Tic Talk

Common Misconceptions, Natural Approaches, and Real Conversations About Tic Disorders

To my boys:

Whit, Wyatt, and Jason

Whit this journey is for you, you are an extraordinary human!

Wyatt and Jason, thank you for always supporting my wacky ideas.

I love you all!

Published by:
Four Eagles Publishing,
Newcastle, NSW, Australia
www.foureaglespublishing.com

A catalog record for this book is available from the National Library of Australia

ISBN: 978-0-6454618-3-1

TABLE OF CONTENTS

FOREWORD

Like a Thief in the Night

A Tic disorder comes along like a thief in the night to steal the peace and joy of your family's existence leaving you feeling scared, alone, and helpless.

Much more than mere words, stories capture the essence of a struggle and show how much of an experience you have had with something. I wrote this book to share with you my struggles of guiding my child through a Tic disorder both from a personal level and from a professional level.

Tics are surprisingly common in children. They can persist to adulthood and evolve if not properly attended to. As a mother, I know too well the pains of having to see your child suffer and wanting so badly to get them back to health. I fully understand the emotions that words cannot possibly describe when it comes to just wanting to have your child back. I went through these experiences for more than six years. I understand the sacrifices, the pains, and the tears that play out and how deeply a mother's love influences all your decisions, including your nutrition and that of your child, as well as the sleepless nights spent worrying about your entire family.

More importantly, I managed to overcome those struggles and nursed my child back to health which is all that mattered and exactly why you are reading this book. My experiences, pains, emotions, trials, research, failures, and successes in helping my son recover from Tics are the main reason I am in the best position to share my experiences with you.

I have written down all my knowledge in the first part of this book and accompanied them with detailed explanations of the solutions, discussing the major factors that influence Tics and how they can be managed. Furthermore, I have put in my ample years of experience as a mother and as a doctor and tried as much as I can to bring all my experiences to you in a comprehensive, simple to understand and compelling book.

This book presents information regarding Tics and Tourette's syndrome. We will explore the myths, the facts, and simple tips that will help you as a parent to reduce the frequency and intensity of Tics to help your child get through the day peacefully. This book offers need-to-know facts that are usually ignored by most doctors, neurologists, and pediatricians, which have an enormous effect on the health of young kids with Tics or Tourette's syndrome.

I am certain you will find this book helpful. Ultimately, I hope you see yourself in my struggles and, through my experiences, draw strength from them and never give up on your child through your journey.

To the improving health of your child,
Dr. Piper Gibson, DFM, AHND, TND, BCDNM

PART 1

Experiencing Tics for The First Time

Chapter 1

Band Aids and Bullshit

This is an intense and emotional story which, if you are reading this, I know you can relate to...

My son's symptoms started long before he had a Tic. When I look back, from the second Whit was born, I can recognize every subtle sign and symptom along the way, and I can see why we ended up where we did. Hindsight is a kick in the ass that way!

Whit was born by C-section, and I can remember the cold room and the window where the sun was just beginning to rise. I remember the pressure of them trying to pull him out, it took three doctors to get the job done. That day the very first thing that the nurses said was, "He has low blood sugar. We must give him sugar water." I was still laying there being stitched up, was pumped full of morphine, and my head was spinning. I didn't have a second to think that they should have brought him to me for breast milk. The best way to prevent low blood sugar in babies is to provide them with breast milk. Since Whit was born via C-section that also means he missed all of the essential microorganisms in the birth canal and the very first thing he was exposed to was sugar. Sugar is inflammatory, it has no nutritional value, and it causes inflammation. Breast milk is full of antibodies and high levels of secretory immunoglobulin A (SIgA) to protect your baby's gut, plus it helps to kill off viruses and bacteria. We were off to a great start!

He was jaundiced from birth, and we had to have bilirubin lights brought into our home so that he could lay under the lights every day. That lasted for almost two weeks. That constant exposure to artificial lights cannot possibly be suitable for a baby's circadian rhythm, which helps to regulate sleep, and this child did not sleep.

I also noticed that Whit had very runny stools, and his diaper was frequently streaked with blood. When we asked the pediatrician, she said, "He must be allergic to your breast milk. You have to give him formula." My brain was reeling as I wondered to myself, "Humans have been on the planet for millions of years, how many babies are allergic to breast milk...?" That started my first research project and what I found was that it wasn't necessarily my breastmilk, but the dairy proteins that I was consuming that could be affecting him. I decided to stop eating dairy the entire time I breastfed him.

Around two months of age, he began getting frequent ear infections. He would wake up in the middle of the night with fluid seeping out of his ears. Whit never slept for long periods at a time, and I was exhausted and stressed. My husband would sleep with him elevated on his chest just to get some relief. I felt like we were at the pediatrician's office every five minutes. By the time he was seven months old, we had probably done eight rounds of antibiotics and at this point, he had to get ear tubes to prevent ear infections. However, they did not seem to make any difference, and we continued to use antibiotics throughout the first year of his life. We now know how damaging antibiotic use is to our gut and our microbiome. Babies are born with very permeable intestines, and all of that excessive antibiotic use continues to damage his gut to this day.

When he was an infant, he also experienced massive reflux, so back to the pediatrician we went where we were prescribed Prilosec. I was giving a child, only months old, at least two prescription medications at any one time. Studies show that acid blockers are only meant to be taken for a short period and that they damage our ability to digest our food and absorb nutrients. I was giving him a dropper or two, daily, of acid blockers as advised by the pediatrician.

Here we were with a brand-new baby on antibiotics and acid blockers who had already had surgery to prevent more ear infections. All the signs were there that something was wrong, but nobody could pinpoint the cause, and I didn't know any better.

When he was nine months old, I got pregnant with my second child, and my milk dried up. The pediatrician said, "Soy formula is best because we know he has issues with dairy." The soy formula caused him to projectile vomit like a scene from *The Exorcist.* The doctor always had the same response, "Give him more Prilosec, it's just reflux."

Even after Whit was a year old and started eating more solid food, he still never slept well. He would not nap during the day and at night he would sleep for only a few hours and wake up restless. My husband worked the graveyard shift and slept during the day. We had a newborn and Whit had chronic health issues. I was one exhausted mama.

Whit spoke well, and he spoke early, so he seemed to be on a fantastic developmental path. He was also very active and was climbing stairs before he could even walk. When we took him to the pediatrician, he was the perfect height and weight, so we felt that there wasn't anything to worry about.

I will honestly tell you that by the time he was one, he could easily order Chicken McNuggets® at the McDonald's drive-through. I know that probably horrifies you but, we didn't know any better. My husband and I were both healthy, fit, and from athletic backgrounds, and, on paper, our children were healthy. Our playdates revolved around trips to Burger King and McDonald's, where we would have lunch, and the kids would play in the playground. With a husband working crazy shifts, we ate a lot of fast food and processed easy-to-prepare food. I was an expert at slinging chicken nuggets into the microwave and whipping up Kraft macaroni and cheese.

Around the time he turned two, Whit started having significant meltdowns, uncontrollable fits, and moodiness. Nothing would soothe him. We chalked it up to the terrible twos... and then the terrible threes. He also became violent, especially towards his brother. My husband and I had planned a trip to Jamaica for our tenth anniversary and my mom came to stay with the boys. While we were away Whit grabbed his brother and tried to pound his head into a wall. Freaking out, my mother called me, and I made an appointment with our doctor for when we got home. He would also kick, hit, and bite other kids. When I addressed this issue with our doctor she said, "It's just his age, it's normal." Since he was my first child, I didn't think much of his fits of rage.

When he was four, the eye blinking started. I know now that the blinking was his very first Tic. We took him to the doctor and were told it was just allergies. Lo and behold, they prescribed Claritin and Zyrtec to help with his dry eyes and allergies. Here we were with yet another prescription to put a Band-Aid on whatever was going on deeper inside his body.

Just more Band-Aids and bullshit!

At one point, I noticed that Whit had bumps all over the front of his chest, and when we addressed it with the pediatrician, she told us it was keratosis, and there was nothing we could do about it but "ignore it". This was the first time a doctor told us to ignore a symptom.

He chronically complained of tummy aches, and headaches, and that he simply didn't feel right. Doctors told us that this was normal because children's nerves start to reach full growth potential around age three or four, and they all start to complain about how they feel.

I had joined a mother's group in the new city we moved to, and some of the other mothers disliked me because they felt that my child did not behave. They saw his meltdown mode and refused to let him play with their kids. It was heartbreaking because, at this point, I was already starting to feel like there was nobody who understood, and there was no support. I could not take my kids to Target without him having a complete meltdown. Often, I would have to abandon the cart in the aisle and leave. I was that mom who was yelling at her kids through clenched teeth because I was exhausted. I didn't know how to get my child to behave.

Somewhere between the age of four and six, he started sniffing and mildly clearing his throat. We didn't think much of it. We chalked it up to allergies.

He was six when we experienced our very first massive Tic episode. We had gone on a trip to Disneyland and overindulged in all the amazingness from donuts to chocolate milk. The day after we returned, he woke up blinking and jerking his neck. We were terrified; we had no clue what was going on. By the end of the day, his neck and head hurt, and he could not control his movement. My husband videotaped it. We immediately got an appointment with the pediatrician who diagnosed an ear infection, prescribed some antibiotics, and sent us on our way. Ten days later, when the antibiotics had not done anything for his symptoms, we were back at the pediatrician's office. This time the pediatrician said, "I think he has a transient neurological Tic; I will send you to the neurologist." That sounded scary and I was scared! ***What is wrong with his brain?*** The pediatrician said, "It's probably nothing, he will grow out of it. I would like to see what the neurologist says," and he sent us on our way.

What the hell was a transient neurological Tic? My husband and I started reading books and scouring Dr. Google for information on Tics, while we waited for our neurologist appointment. We found out that a transient Tic is a Tic that lasts for a short period and can include vocal and motor Tics. When we had our first appointment with the neurologist, the doctor said, "No need for an MRI, I think he needs a good spanking! Ignore it and he will grow out of it." He was six years old and could not control his bodily movements. I was floored and confused. I sat there staring at him with my mouth hanging open. I looked from the doctor to my husband and all I could think was, ***why on earth are we going to spank him? He cannot control his body and we are supposed to spank it out of him?*** This, by far, was the worst medical advice we had ever received.

Over time, his Tic symptoms only worsened. Not only did he now have the motor Tics of the jerking and the blinking, but he also started to have more intense vocal Tics like chronic throat clearing. We couldn't go to a movie or out in public without people staring because this little boy could not control his movements or his noises. It was breaking my heart, but still, no answers were to be found anywhere.

By this point, it was my goal to learn everything I possibly could about Tics. I felt like there had to be an answer out there somewhere. We read pub-med studies and nothing on YouTube provided a positive outlook on Tics and Tourette's. Maybe, eventually, he would grow out of it. Everything out there says ignore it.

But I knew deep down in my mama soul that there was something deeper going on.

We spent thousands of dollars on tests, doctor visits, medicines, and supplements. We visited doctor after doctor who told us to ignore it and that he would grow out of it. He was put on tons of prescriptions, and nothing worked. We were offered more medications with scary side effects when the first prescriptions didn't work. In total, we saw eight different doctors and tried ten prescriptions.

The situation at school was so bad that I pulled my kids out to homeschool them. We spent six years visiting doctors and specialists, and nothing ever changed. I wanted to pull my hair out, I was beyond frustrated and overwhelmed. I was scared and heartbroken when I thought of what Whit's future would be like.

I broke down in rooms full of other mothers, begging for their prayers because I did not know what else to do. I spent many nights crying into my pillow and screaming at God to give us some answers. I was beginning to feel like maybe this was just his lot in life, and he would be forced to struggle with it forever.

As a mom, I spent hours, months, and years of research to try and figure out where we were headed. I had officially become a mega researcher, and I started to educate myself on everything from diet to genetics.

The elementary school called frequently, and they were frustrated because he would eat the school lunch, drink soy milk, and then vomit everywhere. We went to see an allergist who refused to test my son for food allergies. "There has to be a connection to food," I said. He responded, "Nope, he doesn't have the typical food allergy symptoms like swelling of the lips or tongue." Instead, he found it entirely appropriate to prescribe six medications at once. He had the nerve to tell me, "I wouldn't worry about giving Whit this many medications, I would give these meds to my own kids." I immediately went for another opinion with an ear, nose, and throat doctor who told us, "Take him off all of those meds, they won't help and it's way too many."

I began to seek alternative methods that might help my son. I continued reading everything I could get my hands on. One day my best friend called me up and said she had read an article in the newspaper about a little girl in town who had had similar symptoms and that there was an alternative allergist who had helped her. I immediately picked up the phone and scheduled an appointment. This doctor was excellent and was one of the major players in helping us get on the right path. At the first appointment, she took one look at him and said, "He's allergic to dairy, and gluten; plus, he has candida overgrowth. I can tell by looking at him but let's run some tests." She tested Whit for food allergies and food sensitivities, and the allergist was completely correct in her diagnosis. Whit was allergic to dairy, wheat, gluten, peanuts, eggs, and soy. These also happen to be the top six inflammatory foods. Once again, another medication: nystatin, short-term, to help with candida overgrowth.

At this point, we began to see some improvement in the Tics, but they did not completely go away. When we cut out things like peanuts, he immediately stopped clearing his throat. We did continue to struggle with some of the Tics and several of the behavioral symptoms. At one point, she diagnosed him with sensory processing disorder and sent us for occupational therapy. He also struggled with low concentration and dysgraphia.

Although we started to see some improvements, what we were doing with the alternative allergist was just not enough and we continued to struggle. She suggested that maybe he had an MTHFR (methylenetetrahydrofolate reductase) gene mutation, and she ran a test for that. He did have a homozygous mutation, and she felt that he needed some glutathione, a multivitamin, and a digestive enzyme. As I started to research genetics, she told me that I had gone above and beyond her scope of practice, and she encouraged me to find someone else who specialized in the areas that I was researching.

One day, my sister called me and said that she had been in a Facebook group where a woman spoke about a doctor she had seen in Austin, Texas, who had changed her son's life. At that point we felt like we had tried everything and didn't have answers, so we were going to give it a whirl. I called and made an appointment, but there was no room for six months.

At our first appointment, it was suggested that we run a complete nutrigenomic panel on my son. Nutrigenomics is the science of genetics and nutrition. After our meeting, my husband thought the doctor could be a snake oil salesman, and he didn't have a lot of confidence in the things that he was recommending. However, I was hopeful! Once we got Whit's results, we would have a follow-up to come up with a personalized plan for him. Based on Whit's genetics, we knew he was predisposed to chronic aggressive inflammation. He was not a good methylator, he was sensitive to glutamates, and he needed additional glutathione and vitamin D. He also had some nutritional deficiencies that needed to be addressed.

We were blown away in the first 30 days by the changes that happened in our son. His Tic symptoms started to subside, and his behavior and sleep improved immensely. We were shocked that this was working for him!

During this time, I started to go back to school and relearn everything I thought I knew about health and wellness. I became a Certified Functional Diagnostic Nutrition Practitioner®. Nutrigenomics has been so successful for us, and I asked my son's new doctor to train me in the protocol they used with Whit so that I could also share it with others.

This journey has forever changed the course of our lives and, although the struggle was intense, we have seen the light at the end of the tunnel. I fully believe that individual health and wellness are the future, and the future is now. I have gone on to get my Doctorate in Holistic Nutrition, Functional Medicine, Traditional Naturopathy, and become a Board-Certified Doctor of Natural Medicine (an Alternative Practitioner; I am not a physician). I use a step-by-step, whole-body approach when working with my clients to help reduce inflammation, spectrum disorders, ADD/ADHD (attention deficit hyperactivity disorder), Tics/Tourette's, auto-immune, gastrointestinal problems, methylation deficiency, and genetic SNPs (single nucleotide polymorphisms–AKA broken genes). My focus is on real food nutrition, functional lab testing, and genetics so that you can fuel your brain, body, and being.

Had I known then what I know now, I would have done things so much differently. Somehow the journey we have been on was meant for us. It was a guide to show us a different way of life. We needed to look deeper; we needed to look under the hood and outside the box. We were disconnected from our bodies and following the Reductionist Theory (more on that in Chapter 3) of health didn't help. This kept anyone from connecting the dots for a very long time. A diagnosis did not give us answers, it only gave us a label, and we could choose to live with that label or overcome it. There is hope in the journey, and there are answers out there if you decide to step out of the box and find them.

Chapter 2

Most People Get Tics All Wrong

Suddenly, your child is blinking their eyes uncontrollably, or perhaps they are jerking their head from side to side and when you ask them to stop, they tell you they can't. You start thinking, *what is wrong with my child?* There is nothing "wrong" with your child, they simply have a Tic, and the good news is, your child can return to "normal".

Tics are a common health challenge faced by children but may also be present in adults. However, they are an area misunderstood by parents and most of the conventional medical community. Tics can originally start with something as simple as excessive blinking of the eyes, which usually goes misdiagnosed as allergies. However, over time, if not addressed as it ought to be, Tic symptoms can become worse. Typically, Tics occur for the first time around age five, however many silent symptoms like constipation, ear infections, tummy aches, mood swings, poor handwriting, and even sleep issues get written off.

What Are Tics?

The dictionary describes a Tic as "habitual spasmodic contraction of the muscles, most often in the face".

I think the dictionary is wrong... it's not that simple to explain and even less simple to experience.

Tics can come on suddenly and may include constant muscle movements, vocal noises, throat clearing, and uncontrollable jolts of the body. Tics occur at random and are likely to occur several times within a day. Oftentimes, Tics are difficult to control, and kids are likely to explain by saying that they feel the urge to move in a certain way or they might just explode. Most people will tell you that the major sign or explanation of a Tic is that they do not feel as though they are in control of their own bodies.

Classifications of Tics

There are two major types of Tics: motor and vocal.

Vocal Tics: Vocal Tics involve making noise with your mouth or vocal cords. Interestingly, vocal Tics are sounds that are common and that people are familiar with. Examples are:

- Whistling
- Bird or animal noises
- Coughing
- Throat clearing
- Barking
- Grunting
- Sniffing
- Screeching
- Obsessive phrases or phrase repetition

Motor Tics: Motor Tics are the repetitive movements of some parts of your body. Since the condition is common in children, you might notice the following changes in your child:

- Face scrunching
- Nose wrinkling
- Shoulder shrugging
- Eye blinking
- Rubbing hands or feet together
- Repetitive or obsessive touching
- Head twitching or jerking
- Kicking
- Jumping
- Banging
- Flapping

Most times, Tics are broken down into two categories: simple and complex. A simple Tic is a process that involves a single action, while a complex Tic involves several actions or might be a blend of a single vocal and/or a motor Tic.

Let's put things into perspective.

Tics can be defined as transient or chronic. Most children are affected by transient conditions with their symptoms lasting for only a few days or months.

Some children experience chronic Tic conditions and their symptoms last for more than a year in most cases. It is important to note that chronic Tics change from time to time as they can easily switch from vocal to motor or from complex to simple Tics.

Although most Tics are diagnosed as transient, they share the same attributes as those with chronic conditions. For instance, people with chronic motor Tics who experience head/neck twitches over time may see their symptoms develop into other actions such as eye blinking or throat clearing.

A condition known as Tourette's syndrome (TS) is often diagnosed when a child or adult experiences both vocal and motor Tics, which last for more than a year. Close to 138,000 children are said to be diagnosed with Tourette's syndrome in the US alone. The data reveals that boys are four times more affected than girls. The data also shows that it is frequent in younger people aged between 12 to 17 compared to those aged six to 11.

Statistics have also shown that at least 79% of those diagnosed with TS have been diagnosed with repetitive mental health issues and other neurodevelopmental conditions. Furthermore, at least 64% have been diagnosed with ADHD, 43% with behavioral or conduct problems, 40% with anxiety, 36% with depression, and 28% with a developmental delay impeding the child's ability to learn.

As a parent, I know you feel afraid, confused, overwhelmed, and concerned about your child's future. I promise that by the end of this book you will be armed with the information you need to help your child to reduce the symptoms they are struggling with.

Chapter 3

Tics Are Not Purely Neurological

There are certain conventional approaches and schools of thought that believe that Tics are purely neurological. This theory is referred to as the Reductionist Theory. As a result, a Tic is considered a complex condition that comes from and affects only the brain. As time goes on, more research has shown that this is untrue.

In recent years, the American Pediatrics Association has reported that there has been an increase in the level of Pediatric Autoimmune Neuropsychiatric Syndrome (PANS) and Pediatric Autoimmune Neuropsychiatric Disorder Associated with Streptococcal Infections (PANDAS) diagnoses among children. According to the survey carried out by PANDAS network, at least one in every 200 children is affected by PANDAS/PANS. PANDAS causes neuropsychiatric symptoms, specifically obsessive-compulsive disorder (OCD) or Tics. Oftentimes, PANDAS patients test positive for recent streptococcal infection, including strep throat, peri-anal strep, or scarlet fever.

In the same vein, PANS is a diagnosis given to children who have a unique set of symptoms, including obsessions/compulsions and Tics. Although a lot of them are incorrectly diagnosed with OCD. Ultimately, the sudden emergence of symptoms is a sign of PANS.

Most of the children diagnosed with PANDAS and PANS experience symptoms such as depression, anxiety, irritability, and difficulty with schoolwork. Although strep has a direct relationship with PANDAS, the cause of PANS remains unknown. In fact, a series of research has shown that PANS can be caused by infections, food, metabolic issues, environmental factors, and other inflammatory influences.

Another common term used is Pediatric Acute Autoimmune Encephalitis (PAAE). Encephalitis, which is caused by a viral infection, is the swelling of the brain. This way, the terms PANS/PANDAS and PAAE are again linked, although they both have additional symptoms beyond those of strep infection or OCD.

The following is a list of PANS/PANDAS that will help show how far your child has progressed with the disorder:

- Unusual movements such as Tics or twitches, especially around the eyes or mouth. They can also be diagnosed as neurological Tics.
- Staring spell
- Handwriting difficulties
- Eating disorders
- Separation anxiety
- Irritability or outbursts of rage
- OCD symptoms (e.g., fear of contamination, needing things to be "just so" or in specific places, etc.)

There are different degrees of PANS/PANDAS. As a result, symptoms might be difficult for even your doctor to see or diagnose. Therefore, it is essential that you know these symptoms and how to deal with them immediately as they arise. When any of these symptoms pop up it can be essential to contact your pediatrician to conduct a strep test.

From my experience as a practitioner and a parent, I am certain that Tics are not just something that has to do solely with the brain alone. Ultimately, a Tic is a symptom telling you that your body is not in the best state of balance. Tics are like the check engine light that shows on your dashboard, as a healthy body does not show symptoms that depict illness in this way. When something is wrong with your car, the check engine light gives you a warning, it's time to get your car to the shop. In the same vein, Tics are the child's body screaming for help. A Tic is not the problem, it is a sign that there is a problem.

When we equate what is going on with your child to a neurological issue, we are missing a huge piece of the puzzle. Every system, organ, tissue, and cell in the body is connected, and blaming it all on the brain leaves valuable information unexplored.

Tics are just one of the symptoms. Tics, along with brain fog, poor memory, lack of focus, mood swings, constipation, panic attacks, and even depression, are all signs that something is out of balance inside your child's body. Tic disorders are not neurological issues; they are physical imbalances affecting the brain. Something has triggered this event, and the investigation into figuring it out must begin.

The Conventional Approach

I know that up to this point you have asked your doctor a million questions about your child's health. You want to know what is going on and how you can help them feel amazing and in control. In fact, when Tics are involved, and when

ADHD, anxiety, and OCD begin to play out, we start to panic. In most cases, you are likely to leave the doctor's office more confused than when you came in the door. I get it and we have been through it all. In most cases, the conventional approach does not look beyond the outward symptoms. Most Tic diagnoses are given merely by observation and nothing more. Think back to your car and the check engine light. If your mechanic came out and simply looked at your car and said, "Meh, ignore it," you would be furious!

Let me ask you, "Why is this acceptable for our children? Why are we not looking deeper?" As a parent, we should always ask, "Why?" We want to know what the root of the problem is, not slap a Band-Aid on it.

Oftentimes, the typical response for Tics is, "Just give it time; they will outgrow it." "We don't know, but don't worry about it," and that response seems to be the gold standard. So, this begs an important question, "Why take your child to see the doctor over and over?" Most parents feel that they need to see a doctor because they have grown up with the conventional medicine idea that the doctor will fix them. We see the doctor, we get a pill, we go home, and we feel better. When it comes to chronic illnesses like Tics, this approach doesn't work. Another reason why we do this is that we all carry health insurance, and we want our insurance to cover our medical visits. We end up going back to the doctor time after time and we leave without answers. It is what is referred to as the cycle of trial and error. Go to the doctor and get a pill. When that doesn't work, return, and repeat, repeat, repeat. If you ask me, it's a form of insanity, doing the same thing over and over and expecting a different result. According to research, it has been noted that at least 25% of children in the United States are on one medication, while 10% of children are on more than one prescription.

Oftentimes, our children are given drugs based on an observational diagnosis without any laboratory tests being considered. Why is that? Why did our allergist outrightly refuse to order food allergy testing for my son because the symptoms didn't "seem like it"? Instead, he gave us six prescriptions before sending us on our way. Then another doctor told us, "Oh my God, I would never give my kid six prescriptions at once. Plus, they won't do any good."

Are you prepared to go a little further?

Prescribing medications is how physicians are trained. Medical schools do not provide nutrition training or lab testing above the standard blood test. They do, however, spend hours teaching that there's a pill for every ill and what prescription best fits your child's symptoms. Conventional medical training teaches how to use pharmaceutical drugs by using biochemistry in addition to clinical diagnosis. There isn't a pill that will fix the root cause. They will however cover up the symptoms, just like a Band-Aid. Conventional medicine is taught to suppress symptoms with pharmaceutical medications, not get rid of them. This type of medicine does not address the real problem but instead diagnoses the symptoms and tells you that there is no hope for a cure unless they write a prescription. This approach ignores most preventable diseases by pushing pills like statins to lower cholesterol or immunosuppressants to address things like autoimmune issues. Conventional medicine is just that, a pharmacological approach to healthcare. Conventional means it's not holistic, and it will only treat the symptoms and never get to the root cause of illness. Sadly, conventional medicine ignores nutrition, which is an important aspect of preventative care, getting healthy, and staying healthy.

In some instances, prescriptions can offer more profit. Doctors were trained to give medications and not order the right amount of testing because it is a lot easier, more profitable to the establishment, and less invasive. How do doctors make money by prescribing medications? Doctors will most likely make money from medications by writing scripts for them. When the patient pays a co-payment, the doctor's office makes more cash flow (in addition to insurance payments, Medicaid reimbursements, etc.). This is one of the reasons why doctors prescribe medications even when they may not be needed. It also explains why many doctors do not order lab testing. This will also keep you coming back for more, and the doctor will get to bill your insurance for return visits. If you need a refill many times, you will be required to make an appointment where your doctor will evaluate you and give you another script. Prescribing a medication can mean big business for doctors, hospitals, pharmaceutical companies, and the medical profession. Conventional treatments are given to patients even though they don't work because of a hyper fixation on profits. Conventional treatments are often more expensive than alternative therapies, which also contributes to profitability. Conventional treatments frequently provide only temporary relief; however, when it comes to the bottom line, writing a prescription wins. This is how the conventional system is set up, and things don't seem to be changing anytime soon. Conventional medical treatments include surgical procedures, medications, and other physical methods to treat disease. Conventional medicine is a multi-billion-dollar industry that continues to grow with the increasing number of people using conventional medical treatment.

Insurance organizations possess a lot of authority. Health insurance companies have always used their powers to influence the actions of physicians. They can tell the doctors the tests they cover and how much they are willing to reimburse them. This implies that the doctor will be forced to use an in-office lab, followed by prescriptions that might shape our healthcare system.

The advertisement of drugs on TV makes the acceptance of pills and drugs more appealing as a solution for most health problems. Therefore, patients appear before the doctor with a notion that supports the use of drugs and their characteristics that have been described on TV. The doctor's job is a lot easier when you show up with what you want instead of what you need. Interestingly, the US is one of the few countries that allow the media to directly advertise prescriptions and medications to the public.

Just like adults, kids in the US are given drugs for chronic ailments. The fact of the matter is that functional lab tests have been shown to be more effective in the long run than medications or prescriptions. Functional lab tests have proven to be of great help in identifying the root cause, and the causes of the symptoms, and creating a solution through specific recommendations such as major lifestyle adjustments. Through this, you have data to back up what's happening with your child's health and take control of it.

Ultimately, this section is not an endorsement for kids to stop taking their medications or to bad mouth the conventional approach. Doctors are necessary if you break an arm or have a heart attack; you need them for acute care. It's long-term chronic care that fails when it comes to conventional medicine. This is a reminder that there are other options out there.

Stress Factors

All diseases have a beginning, but conventional doctors make Tic disorders seem like they just appear out of thin air, something that just comes on without any cause. They do not consider how toxins, nutrient deficiencies, or infections impact each child differently. Stress caused by certain triggers can start changing brain chemistry long before these symptoms become apparent, making it nearly impossible to pinpoint why the Tic appeared NOW. Tics are not purely neurological in nature but are the body's way of communicating that something is wrong.

Tics are a symptom, not an illness. Tics are caused by an imbalance in the body, and they can be changed or undone with specific alterations to diet, and lifestyle habits, and through rebalancing the body systems using natural approaches.

At some point, most children experience triggering events that can be caused by many factors such as stress, nutrient deficiency, food sensitivities, allergies, live vaccines, toxin exposure, infections, illness, and even growth. Tics may show up in a child who has been exposed to toxicants such as heavy metals (from dental amalgams), pesticides, herbicides, and other toxic chemicals from food/air/water pollution, environmental pollution, including mold exposure from damp basements to water damage in homes from natural disasters like hurricanes, typhoons, and floods.

Tics may also surface with chronic low-grade infections like viruses or bacteria in the gut, brain, or other areas of the body. Low-grade infections can be considered an underlying stressor that goes undetected. The conventional approach does not usually look deep enough to sniff out if an underlying infection is even present in a child with a Tic disorder. Although we know from PANS/PANDAS research those underlying infections can have an impact on Tics. That research is still not taught in most conventional medical schools, and I have come across many parents whose physicians tell them that PANS/PANDAS is not real.

Tics may also be a sign of imbalanced hormones, which are often the byproduct of a poor diet. Tics can also be related to something as simple as neck tension from poor posture or the consequence of spending too much time with electronics, including TV, gaming (video games), smartphones, and tablets. Tics can also be a sign that there is an imbalance in the nervous system due to trauma, stress, anxiety, emotional distress, including Post Traumatic Stress Disorder (PTSD) or depression, and even spiritual unrest like unhealed grief/loss/trauma.

Tics can often occur when there is an imbalance in the body, and it simply tells us that something needs to change before they become more serious symptoms and health problems arise later down the road.

Tracking your child's triggers can be difficult and requires a very mindful and vigilant effort. Once you've become aware of the "triggers" for your child's Tic disorder, you can begin the process of rebalancing by creating a healthy environment for your child and family. This can help everyone in the home and helps to ease anxiety and stress levels, which is a key factor in reducing Tic symptoms.

Here are some of the things that might continue to spur your child's Tic symptoms:

Infection: Tics are increased during cold and flu season when your child is exposed to new viruses. A history of ear infections can be a cause of OCD and other neurobehavioral disorders as well as Tic disorders. Ear infections are usually triggered by dairy sensitivity, which links back to food. Hidden infections like protozoa, candida, and other bacterial/microbial overgrowths in the gut can also impact your child's symptoms.

Toxins: Tics are also triggered by exposure to pollutants in the air from wildfires, car exhausts, cleaning products in the home, air fresheners, scented candles, scented laundry detergent, dryer sheets, or second-hand smoke. There are other potent toxins in the home: the body care products our children use daily, such as shampoo/conditioner, creams, soaps, and deodorants /antiperspirants. Not to mention what our children are eating and drinking out of, like non-stick cookware and plastics. Tic disorder can also be spurred by drinking well water, living near a major highway or industrial area that releases chemical fumes (e.g. dry cleaners), usage of pesticides (or having pets exposed to them). Tics can also be caused by mercury amalgam fillings and high levels of aluminum found in vaccines. Tics may also be prevalent in children who have been vaccinated for the flu which contains thimerosal (mercury derivative) given during pregnancy at 28 weeks' gestation through to six months of age.

Food sensitivity: Gluten sensitivity and celiac disease have been linked with many neurological syndromes, including ADHD, autism spectrum disorders, dyslexia, schizophrenia, and epilepsy. Many other food sensitivities can be triggers for Tics, including dairy, eggs, and other grains such as corn or rice. Tics can also be triggered by an intolerance to sugar and artificial sweeteners/colorings in foods or drinks.

Lyme disease: Tics are also common symptoms associated with Lyme disease. They may also occur along with other neurological syndromes linked to Lyme disease, such as Bell's palsy, encephalopathy/encephalitis, meningitis, neck stiffness with hearing loss, and aphasia (inability to speak or comprehend speech). Lyme disease is not just passed on from tick bites. It is possible to get this infectious illness through sexual contact and blood transfusions, as well as in-utero exposure to mothers who were infected during pregnancy.

Toxic mold: Mold in the home or workplace can be toxic and cause Tic disorders. Toxins in the body from mold exposure include mycotoxins, aflatoxin B1, trichothecene, volatile organic compounds (VOCs), and Stachybotrys chartarum (SC) toxins, which affect not only your neurological health but also your immune system. Tics are one of the most common presenting issues linked to toxic mold illness, according to Dr. Shoemaker, MD. Tics associated with mold illness take longer than a few weeks or months to resolve and often wax and wane over many years, depending on the level of contamination and type of toxin(s). Mold Toxin Immune Load – toxins from mold affect both the immune system and neurological pathways leading to Tics. Tachycardia (high heart rate), poor ability to concentrate, mood swings, etc., all symptoms present in Lyme disease, may also present in those with Tic disorders.

Nutrient deficiencies: Tic disorders can also represent nutrient deficiencies and can be linked to an imbalance in neurotransmitters, hormones, minerals, essential fatty acids, and growth factors/peptides. Tics may also result from genetic susceptibility to nutrient deficiency, impacted by a lack of key nutrients needed for proper brain development and function.

Liver toxicity: Tics may represent liver toxicity caused by medication prescribed by conventional MDs who do not understand the role of nutrition and detoxification in health. Tics are often seen in children being treated with medications, like ADHD drugs, which damage the liver. Tics may also be seen in children with behavioral issues who have been prescribed Tylenol, which is toxic to the liver.

Seasonal allergies: Pollen, dust, grass, weeds, and dander may also be a trigger for Tics. Often Tic symptoms occur with other allergic symptoms like runny nose, watery eyes, and skin rash in response to pollen exposure. Tic disorders are found at high incidence in patients with allergies and asthma.

Anxiety, emotional trauma, and unresolved stress: Tics may also be seen as a way for the nervous system or brainstem to cope with anxiety, stress, or fear in children who suffer from some sort of emotional trauma or stress. Anxiety triggers Tics by causing inflammation and neurotoxicity/damage to the brain. Often kids will Tic less when they learn ways to manage their emotions, through counseling, meditation, and even deep breathing.

Sensory input: Tics and Tic disorders have very strong connections to sensory input such as iPads, video games, TVs, excessive screen time, WIFI, or other electronics in the home or at school.

Gut issues: Tic disorders tend to develop in kids who have gut imbalances such as leaky gut syndrome (LGS), intestinal infections, parasites, food allergies/sensitivities, or other digestive problems. Children with Tic disorders tend to have some sort of digestive imbalance that causes inflammation in the body. Tics are oftentimes reduced when underlying gut imbalances are resolved.

So, what ties all these triggers together? What is the common factor?

Inflammation! Chronic inflammation is the primary driver of chronic disease and the underlying cause of chronic illnesses. So, if your child has a Tic disorder, it's time to explore where that inflammation is coming from.

Before we dive in, you must understand that inflammation is not simple; inflammation comes in different forms, both necessary for health and harmful at its chronic capacity.

The stressors that we talked about in the previous chapter can all lead to chronic inflammation.

Inflammation is an integral part of your immune response and the first line of defense for your body against harmful stimuli like germs and toxins.

But inflammation, as with all things in life, is not black or white; inflammation can be necessary but also harmful, which means that a specific type of inflammation must be dealt with accordingly (more on inflammation later).

When you get sick or twist your ankle, your immune system goes to work; inflammation in this case is a good thing. For example, you experience a fever or redness and swelling for a few days, but after a few days, you feel better. This is a particular type of inflammation called acute inflammation.

Acute inflammation saves lives when it fights off an infection or injury, but inflammation becomes the real problem if you live in this state chronically throughout your life. This chronic inflammation, also known as systemic inflammation, is caused by chronic stress, food sensitivities/ intolerances/ sensitivity to chemicals, imbalance in the microbiome (good bacteria–bad bacteria ratio), toxicity, and environmental factors. When we are exposed to certain triggers, the body produces small proteins called cytokines. These cytokines facilitate the response of the body to threats and can be measured and used to assess inflammation levels in the body (Chang et al., 2010).

It is evident from looking at study after study that chronic inflammation leads to chronic disease.

Are Tics a chronic disease? In my opinion, yes! Let's break down the word disease: a condition that prevents the body or mind from working correctly. When your child is experiencing Tics, their body is in a state of DIS-ease. When you are healthy and symptom-free, your body is at ease. A Tic disorder is an apparent symptom of a body that is not at ease. A 2019 study connects chronic inflammation and immune dysregulation to the increase of pediatric-onset obsessive-compulsive disorder (OCD) and Tic disorders such as Tourette's syndrome (TS). Chronic diseases, whether autoimmune conditions like Lupus, asthma, or even mental health issues, can all be linked back to inflammation.

Your immune system and neurological system are connected, and when your immune system is always turned on, we can see the impact on the neurological system (the brain). For example, inflammation in the brain may be linked to underlying infections in the gut.

We know that the number one cause of inflammation from food sensitivity is wheat gluten, followed by dairy. So, if you introduce gluten around age one and Tics start to show up around age four or five, it's possible that gluten could be *part* of the cause. Also, as gluten and other stressors break down the gut, we may see more gut issues that impact the brain.

However, chronic inflammation can be caused by many more factors that you will want to consider. Toxins, heavy metals, nutrient deficiency, and underlying infections can contribute to inflammation as well. We know that strep infections are tied to PANDAS diagnosis, and other underlying conditions like Lyme can cause PANS.

Genetic predisposition may also contribute to inflammation. For example, if you are genetically predisposed to chronic inflammation and experience a triggering event, your genes may be playing a role here.

There are many moving parts and pieces of the puzzle. Tic disorders are multilayered, and it may not always be apparent why they are happening. Virtually every chronic neurological condition has inflammation at its core, which then manifests into other symptoms.

This is such an oversimplification of what inflammation is and how it affects your child's Tic disorder. Learning about inflammation was a game changer for my son's Tics, and I could look at it from a different point of view. Remember that inflammation can be caused by many more factors that need to be investigated and not looked at as a singular cause.

Overall, inflammation triggers an aggressive immune system response and neurological reaction. Tics are often attributed to a neurological reaction to inflammation. When we address the root cause of the inflammation, these Tic disorders tend to reduce, resolve, and recover. Tics typically will flare up under times of stress and illness. We will dig deeper into immune response a little later.

Tics are multilayered and you will want to keep in mind that it may not just be one trigger, but many triggers and underlying stressors, that are perpetuating your child's Tics. Tics are commonly misunderstood and misdiagnosed in conventional medical circles. They are the consequence of different underlying conditions that are not typically considered and do not always appear for the first time during childhood or go away on their own. They may be chronic but can resolve over time with the right approach. Tic disorders can remit spontaneously; however, often, Tic disorders will persist if there is a lack of awareness as to what or how to balance the body.

I find it very helpful whenever I am seeing someone new to spend some time looking at the big picture of their health – assessing what has happened thus far with conventional medicine, both naturopathic and conventional treatments, socioeconomic factors, environmental factors, diet (I recommend taking an inventory of everything your child eats), sleep, exercise, screen time, stress levels, etc. Tics can often present in the absence of all other health concerns. I have seen many children who had only one symptom – a Tic. However, it's important to figure out WHY they are experiencing Tics in the first place. Tics may be considered a disease, but they are really a symptom of underlying imbalance.

The Diagnosis Laundry List

As parents, we are always on the lookout for how to stop Tics or Tic disorders however we often don't consider how another diagnosis might be connected to Tics.

Children who suffer from Tic disorders, attention deficit hyperactivity disorder (ADHD), obsessive compulsive disorder (OCD), or sensory processing disorder (SPD) are more likely to have another diagnosis. Tic disorders and other related diagnoses often go hand in hand with each other. A co-diagnosis is when a child has two different diagnoses that go together. Tics may be the most noticeable of these conditions, but they typically accompany one of these three: ADHD, OCD, or SPD. We are going to explore Tic disorders and how they relate to other mental health issues such as ADHD, OCD, SPD, and even autism spectrum disorders (ASD).

Tics may be observed in children diagnosed with ADHD. For example, a child with Tourette's syndrome (TS) accompanied by attention deficits will meet the diagnostic criteria for ADHD. Tic disorder is also comorbid with other impulse control or disruptive behavior disorders such as Conduct Disorder and Oppositional Defiant Disorder which are often seen alongside a diagnosis of ADHD. In addition, Tics can occur alone or co-occur with another neurodevelopmental issue like autism spectrum disorder. Children suffering from Tic disorders usually have more than one motor or vocal Tic, and they may also struggle with mood swings and focus issues.

If your child has more than one diagnosis, I am sure you wonder how they are all connected. For example, Tic disorders, ADHD, SPD, OCD, and ASD, can be connected through similar brain mechanisms.

The connection between Tic disorders, OCD, and SPD...

We know Tics often co-occur with another diagnosis, and they share a common neurological pathway responsible for developing these three conditions, which involves the basal ganglia area in our brains. The basal ganglia play an important role in regulating behavior, cognition, emotions, and movement. Basal ganglia function can be disrupted when our child has a multitude of hidden stressors impacting their bodily functions. You may have heard me say in previous posts that all body systems are connected, and when one system malfunctions, they all become imbalanced.

A disruption in the immune system can lead to Tics, ADHD, and OCD due to allergies, toxins, underlying infections, gut issues, and even food sensitivities. Unfortunately, Tic disorders are often misdiagnosed because of a lack of understanding about what Tics truly represent. Tics usually begin before the age of 18, but they may appear later during adulthood if one has had chronic stressors impacting their body. These chronic stressors (allergies, toxins, underlying infections, gut issues, food sensitivities) can lead to inflammation, leaky gut syndrome, and more.

Tics and OCD often go hand in hand when underlying infections are present, causing inflammation in the brain. PANS and PANDAS are the key diagnoses when these two symptoms suddenly appear. Tic disorders don't just affect children either – many adults struggle with these conditions as well! However, adults will not be diagnosed with PANS or PANDAS because they are specific to the pediatric population. To this end, many adults are left misdiagnosed or untreated because the proper investigation is not being done.

When your child has multiple diagnoses, it is always important to go back to the hidden stressors and inflammation that are most likely at the root of the problem. For example, Tics and OCD are stress-related conditions, so removing the Tic-causing stimuli is crucial in helping your child feel at ease.

Our children's bodies need to recover from the inside out, and we need to remove any obstacles for this process to happen. Children with Tic disorders also have a higher incidence of having several diagnoses or other neurological concerns. I call this the laundry list of symptoms. Your child may have several things going on besides Tics. It is addressing these conditions simultaneously while also addressing underlying causes that really support our children to heal.

Supporting the Entire Body

In my view because Tic disorders are not purely neurological, it is essential to support the entire body in our client care approach. Functional medicine tells us that every system in our body is connected, which is not what we're taught in elementary school during biology class. We have been told that each system in our body is separate. Most of us grew up learning that our digestive system, endocrine system, immune system, and cardiovascular system were all individual working systems. Never once did we learn that they were connected in any way, and this is still the approach that medical schools use today. They still see each system as separate, and that is why we have specialists in every system, organ, bone, and muscle in the body. Therefore, your doctor tells you that diet doesn't matter, or it's all neurological; that's the way they learned, and that's the way they see it.

The functional medicine approach tells us that Tic syndrome is a complex set of symptoms, signs, and behaviors which are associated with biochemical imbalances in the body resulting from internal dysfunction. We know that Tics can be caused by nutritional deficiencies, toxicity, and immune malfunctions and Tic disorders are one of the symptoms of an out-of-balance whole body. Tics represent the fallout from an unhealthy system and addressing them should be part of a holistic approach to health.

Holistic does not mean I'm going to come over and sage your house and rub crystals on you. Holistic simply means relating to, or concerned with, whole or complete systems rather than with the analysis of, treatment of, or dissection into parts. People hear the word holistic and think, "That's for weirdoes" without really knowing that we want to consider your WHOLE child.

As I have mentioned previously, Tics are not only neurological. In fact, Tics can be more than just Tics when other parts of the body begin to show signs that something is wrong. Sadly, one of the features of this epidemic is that Tic disorders are being seen in normally developing children as early as two years old. These kids are then sent off to school where they receive a further dose of immune stress from germs and environmental chemicals along with processed foods and emotional stress.

Tics are part of a bigger cascade, and you don't want to let them get out of control. If you think about an iceberg, you can only see a small fraction of it from the surface, but there is a giant oversized piece of ice just below the surface. When your child is experiencing a Tic, it's likely only the tip of the iceberg. What is going on underneath and pushing the Tic to the surface is even more complex. A functional approach will optimize the system, addressing it not just neurologically, but from every angle, including nutrition, environmental toxins, exercise, stress reduction, hormones/neurotransmitters, etc. This functional approach is investigative and preventative and what I recommend for anyone whose child has a Tic disorder or any other neurological symptom that is just not normal (some examples would be constant headaches, excessive fatigue/sleepiness).

I see Tic disorders from a 30,000-foot perspective. Looking down, we can see all the different factors that might impact a child. I know from experience that Tic disorders go above and beyond the brain, affecting every system in our body. Therefore, it's important to support each system and address those unique needs.

But before we start supporting each system, let's look at what happens when Tics take over the nervous system. The nervous system has two pathways: the sensory pathways (auditory/visual/tactile) and motor pathways (motor cortex to basal ganglia; functional loops between different regions in the brain). When our children experience Tics, signals become disorderly and cause a cascade of disorganization at the functional loop level.

The functional loops need to be organized and regulated by neuro-transmitters such as dopamine, serotonin, GABA, and glutamate. If it is excess or deficient in a particular neurotransmitter, it can contribute to hyperactivity. An example is dopamine an excess of this neurotransmitter is associated with ADHD symptoms, whereas people who have schizophrenia tend to have low concentrations of dopamine in their brains. When the immune system is fired up and activates the nervous system, neurotransmitters are disrupted and result in functional loop deregulation.

Unregulated functional loops lead to functional disruption of the homeostatic systems such as sympathetic, parasympathetic, cardiovascular, pulmonary, gastro-intestinal, endocrinology and immune. Once a functional system is dysregulated, it can negatively influence other systems which are directly linked at the functional loop level. For example, the sympathetic nervous system stimulates sweat production by activating eccrine glands found over most of our bodies but primarily in the palms of hands, soles of feet, and the head; therefore, increased, or reduced activity of the sympathetic nervous system will affect eccrine glands. Stress can also activate or inhibit the hypothalamus in controlling body temperature through sweating (vasodilation).

Microglial cells are the immune system of the brain. They are often found surrounding glutamate receptors and can be activated by the presence of glutamate. Microglial activation can lead to changes in neuronal excitability because there is a chemical change in the environment that they recognize as potentially harmful. When we see an increase in microglial activation in the brain, it causes an overabundance of glutamic acid that excites the brain. When we have an imbalance of GABA and glutamate, it leads to an overstimulation of the excitatory pathways and can lead to a glutamate storm.

Glutamate exposure has been linked to symptoms of ASD, OCD, a whole slew of psychiatric disorders, and chronic pain states. That is not to say that people with Tic disorders have any of those things; however, it means that microglial activity can affect many different brain functions through up-regulation or down-regulation of specific proteins at various synapses.

Although the glutamate storm is causing an excitatory response in the brain, you have to look upstream to figure out what might be triggering this response. Tics seem to be the downstream effect when our brain, nervous, and immune system are stuck in a loop.

Overstimulation of microglia leads to increased expression of pro-inflammatory cytokines, including TNFα, IL-6, IL1β, and others (Yamamoto et al., 2014). The other downstream effect when our immune system is overactive or stuck in a loop is a rise in the level of oxidative stress, which looks like what happens during glutamate toxicity.

It has been said that "with one disease process, you're more likely to have another". That is because of the connection between all of the systems in our bodies. One could say that Tics and Tourette's are immune system problems. But we also need to consider all of the other systems that may be affected by this, such as the neurological and endocrine (hormonal) systems. Overactive microglia can cause an increase in free radical production (Wegner et al., 1999). Overactivation of microglia also causes them to produce more pro-inflammatory chemicals that affect neurotransmitters in the brain, worsening symptoms (Vasilevko et al., 2013).

Comorbidities like OCD are very broad and overlap with many functional conditions. It is likely due to functional dysregulation in several systems of our body. These include the immune system, sympathetic nervous system, parasympathetic nervous system, hypothalamus-pituitary-adrenal axis, autonomic nervous system (ANS), neuroendocrine hormonal regulation (hypothalamus-pituitary-adrenal [HPA] axis), neurotransmitters like dopamine and glutamate pathways that control motor activity, etc.

It is like a domino effect, and once one starts the fall, the rest soon follow. How do we as parents start to stand those dominoes up again and, more importantly, how do we keep them from toppling over again?

PART 2

Get Ready to Kick the Tics

Chapter 4

The Game Plan

Now that we have covered the basics of what Tics are, how they are diagnosed, where they stem from, and how the whole body is impacted, we can finally dig into the process of reducing symptoms naturally. All I have said in the previous chapters will give you a better understanding of what you are dealing with.

When my son was handed a diagnosis in 2011, we felt lost, confused, scared, overwhelmed, and frustrated. We wanted answers to why he suddenly had Tics and what we could do to help. Ignoring it was not a valid option for us and the more Whit struggled, the harder we pressed for answers. As a mom, I wanted someone to hold my hand and walk me through everything I needed to know to get my son back. Sadly, there was no one there. No one had experienced what we were going through and publicly shared what they had learned. No one could provide us with valid answers. No one was able to support us on our journey. That is why I created my own process so that parents like you would have the guidance they needed right from the start.

I wanted a formula! I wanted a step-by-step process with all the tools and resources I needed to help my son. Now I am giving that to you so that you can find success on your journey too.

Are Your Ready to Kick the Tics?

Just like with every formula, there is a process to how things work and how they play out. There are steps that need to be taken to ensure that you get the result that you seek or desire. In the same vein, if you want to help your child recover from Tics or Tourette's syndrome, it is important that you follow several steps. However, it is important that you are resolute and ready to follow through. Going at this half-heartedly will not get you the results you want.

Some of the steps that I will be recommending are:

- Foundational goal setting
- Testing
- Whole foods

- Sugar detox
- Gut health
- Toxins in the home
- Healthy habits
- Resetting the nervous system
- What we changed (D.R.E.S.S)®
- Diet
- Rest
- Exercise
- Supplementation
- Stress reduction
- A personalized plan
- Sample recipes

Chapter 5

Foundational Goal Setting

When you go on a family trip, you don't just hop in the car and drive. You have a plan, and you know where your endpoint is going to be. You know the stops along the way, and the time it will take you to get there. A goal for your child's health requires the same plan. You need all the passengers on board and ready to roll to see results. A key feature to being successful with this is to share the destination of your goal. At the start of this journey, you will want to ask, "What do you want for your child's health?" This really helps you think about what you are doing and why you are doing it. Although it seems straightforward, many parents have not thought through what their goals are when it comes to their children's health.

Oftentimes, health is considered a luxury until it isn't there, then it is considered a necessity. The health of our kids is not always planned, and expectations are not always well written or articulated. As a result, most parents manage what comes their way and settle for what they get if it isn't the worst-case scenario, and they can get by. However, your kid's health should not be a luxury: it is the whole essence of their life. It is vital that you put in the work and take the necessary actions needed to ensure that your wishes and desires for your child translate into reality.

How then can you demand from life the best in terms of health for your child? How can you make the right plans and take the right steps in implementing them? This section is focused on helping you set the right goals, and giving you simple, actionable steps to work on and manage health challenges, such as Tics, through natural processes.

HEALTH GOALS NEED TO BE WRITTEN DOWN

Health goals, particularly those for your child, need to be written down. We are usually only concerned with writing down financial, career, and other types of goals, conveniently excluding health goals. Writing down your health goals helps make your desires and core health values clearer. It makes it easier to break the goals into simple steps that can be followed and makes you accountable in the process. The steps to achieving any dream are usually long and exhausting. Most goals are considered marathons and require consistency to pull through. Writing down your goals opens them up for evaluation and eliminates all forms of could-haves and should-haves. Like all other goals, your foundational goals must be SMART: Specific, Measurable, Action-Oriented, Realistic, and Time Sensitive.

Specific: When setting out on a medical procedure or preparing to undergo a particular process, it is important that you are very clear about what you want. If you are in doubt or unsure, it is important that you try writing out your innermost desires to help you get perspective. For instance, when I started out on all those processes, I had one end in mind – to ensure that all the symptoms of Tics leave my child and that he gets a clean bill of health. This is one of the major things that spurs me and helps me forge ahead. It is important that you clearly explore the "why" so you can effectively plot the "how".

Measurable: The process of evaluation is vital in every single approach or procedure you intend to undergo. For instance, when I visited the doctor that my husband thought was a snake oil salesman – the one who applied the methods that worked so perfectly with Whit, I was able to see the difference that the procedure made within as little as 30 days. It is essential that you measure every process to see how far you have gone and how effective the entire procedure is. You must be able to observe the symptoms and be able to ask your child if he or she feels pain or not. You must be able to observe them and judge if the system is effective. The measurement of your goals will be able to help you forge ahead and reinforce your efforts if they are yielding results or abandon the entire process if it is not working.

Action Oriented: Wishes and intentions have never been enough. Actions are needed to get things done. To get the kind of health you desire, it is important that you put in the work to get results. For instance, you must put in the work in terms of diet, medication, and therapy to help your child overcome the symptoms of Tics.

Realistic: You must also be realistic enough to know that the change you want to see is gradual and will take time to materialize.

Time Sensitive: Famous US author and influencer Napoleon Hill stated that "Goals are dreams with a deadline", and he is right in every way. Putting a timeline on your dream is the key to ensuring that your goals come to fruition. Aside from career and financial goals, it is worth putting a timeline to the health of your child. It is important not to rush processes and practice patience in certain situations, particularly in matters of health. Drugs and therapies are also time-bound, and it is also vital to evaluate the time required to determine their effectiveness.

TOP TIPS FOR SETTING FOUNDATIONAL HEALTH GOALS FOR YOUR CHILD

Be committed to your goals: This means that you will stay true to them as well as the plans and actions mapped out to accomplish them.

Create a plan: It is essential that you create a plan with a specialist or pediatrician to help your child. You must also make sure the plan is practical for you and can yield the best results with your lifestyle, and your child's lifestyle, as well as the ability to create the environment and harness the resources to make it work.

Build an accountability structure: The very idea of helping your child is motivating but when you start out, it is usually challenging. It is easier to say that the child will outgrow the symptoms of the Tics or assume that it's their destiny. It's just too easy to give up when the going gets tough, and you can't see any result. To help you get through, you must get someone who will help keep you focused and engaged in all these processes and hold you accountable, reminding you why you started in the first place. You must ensure it is someone you trust, and who will not give up on you and your child. Through this, you will be able to endure and see through the entire process and achieve your goal regardless of the challenges involved.

Journal Exercise:

Sit with these questions and think about what you ultimately want for your child. I know this process may seem silly but answering these questions can give you some benchmarks and anchors that will help you to stay committed.

Where do you want to see your child's health in 30 days?

Where do you want to see your child's health in 60 days?

Where do you want to see your child's health in six months?

Where do you want to see your child's health in a year?

What short-term steps do you need to take to reach those goals?

What long-term steps do you need to take to reach those goals?

Chapter 6

Testing

Many parents come to me who have no desire to take their child through the conventional approach. Since I do not provide my clients with a diagnosis, many are curious if what their child is experiencing is a Tic.

Tics can be identified through a self-test.

A self-test will only help you get started. It will not give you the data you need to reduce symptoms. That is why we incorporate the test with Comprehensive Neuro-Immune Analysis (CNIA).

This simple self-test can be carried out by honestly answering a series of questions for yourself or your child. The questions are used to check if the traits exhibited match the symptoms of Tic disorder or Tourette's syndrome.

Two of the main research bodies (the National Institute of Neurological Disorders and Stroke and the Yale Global Tic Severity Scale from the Yale Child Study Centre) came up with the tool to help corroborate any other medical findings discovered about the subject. I want you to know that this is not a diagnostic tool, and any deductions made from it must still be corroborated by a medical professional.

TAKE THE TEST

Below are the questions you need to honestly answer to self-test whether you believe you may be experiencing a Tic.

1. Do people mention to you that you make the same sniffing or coughing noise again and again, even when your throat does not tickle?

- ☐ All the time
- ☐ Often
- ☐ Sometimes
- ☐ Rarely
- ☐ Never

2. Do you do familiar hand gestures (such as a thumbs-up) frequently, even at inappropriate times, and you feel like you can't control it?

- ☐ All the time
- ☐ Often
- ☐ Sometimes
- ☐ Rarely
- ☐ Never

3. Do any of these motions (motor Tics) or sounds (vocal Tics) identified in the above two questions result in emotional distress?

- ☐ All the time
- ☐ Often
- ☐ Sometimes
- ☐ Rarely
- ☐ Never

4. Have you been experiencing these Tic-like symptoms for more than one year?

- ☐ Yes
- ☐ No
- ☐ I am not sure

5. During the last month, have you had an increase in the level of oral engagements (verbal Tics) and involuntary movements (motor Tics) for more than half of the entire day?

- ☐ Yes
- ☐ No
- ☐ I am not sure

6. Have you ever been insulted, ignored, embarrassed, or shunned for mimicking what people say even though you didn't intend to but you feel like you couldn't control it?

- ☐ All the time
- ☐ Often
- ☐ Sometimes
- ☐ Rarely
- ☐ Never

7. Do people tell you, or do you realize, that you blink your eyes, twitch your arms, legs, or nose, or jerk your neck for no reason at all?

- ☐ All the time
- ☐ Often
- ☐ Sometimes
- ☐ Rarely
- ☐ Never

8. Do you blurt out random words that are unrelated to the discussion without meaning to?

- ☐ All the time
- ☐ Often
- ☐ Sometimes
- ☐ Rarely
- ☐ Never

If, after taking this self-test, you feel that a diagnosis is an important next step, please see your doctor or neurologist. A self-test is designed to give you only a small clue as to what may be going on. It is your responsibility to decide on the next step for you.

My Approach: Comprehensive Neuro-Immune Analysis

My signature approach is using a technique that I created called Comprehensive Neuro-Immune Analysis® (CNIA).

Although there is not a single test to determine why your child has Tics, there are many functional lab tests that can help us get to the root of the problem. By analyzing data from functional lab testing, we can connect the dots between health history, lab results, and symptoms.

The symptoms our children are experiencing are not normal; they are a check engine light telling you it's time to look under the hood. Your child did not just wake up one day like this; it has been building over time as their little bodies were breaking down on the inside. I always thought that my son just woke up with a Tic, but looking back, I can see the subtle warnings that were showing up more and more frequently.

If you are looking to put all the pieces together, you need to run functional lab tests to look at how the entire body is functioning as a whole unit.

The functional lab testing I use with clients is not found in your average pediatrician's office. In fact, I now teach doctors how to use and interpret many of these tests in their own practice. The following are the key tests I ran with my son and what I use with my clients today.

Stool Pathogen Testing

Stool pathogen testing can be used to assess digestion, microbial imbalances, pathogens, underlying infections, internal inflammation, and toxicity. Hippocrates said, "All disease begins in the gut" and that's not far from the truth!

Over 500 different species of organisms have been found in the human microbiome. Most of them are friendly and they all get along. However, occasionally, you will end up with something that just doesn't belong. That seems to be the case with many of my clients. For every single signal your brain sends to your gut, your gut sends ten signals back to your brain. (The gut can be a little bossy...)

So why is the gut so important?

- Gut Lining: The gut is lined with a mucosal barrier, which acts as an internal second skin to defend against bacteria, viruses, etc.
- The Brain: 95% of serotonin (the hormone that helps you relax) is created in the gut.
- Immunity: 70% of the immune system is found in the gut.
- Nutrients: 90% of vitamins and minerals are absorbed in the small intestine. They are co-factors for enzyme reactions, metabolism, conversion of nutrients and fats, and amino acids (absorbed from digested proteins) which are the precursors for neurotransmitters. Without any of these, we can't function.

What clues are we looking for when using a stool test?

Basically, we are looking for an imbalance of good vs. bad bacteria. Some of the bacteria in our guts are opportunistic and they never miss a chance to take over. When the good bacteria are waning, the opportunistic guys wax on! We are also looking for clues as to how our immune system is functioning. Yes, there are markers in our poo that can tell us what is going on with our immune system. Then there are infections. Viral infections in the gut can often affect the brain. We can also assess digestion, inflammation, and underlying infections. There isn't much we cannot learn from the gut.

A stool pathogen test is just what it sounds like! Poop into a French fry boat, take a sample and send it to the lab. Please don't send me pictures of your child's sample!

Food Sensitivity Testing*

Food sensitivity testing can be used to assess your child's reaction to foods that may be impacting digestion and increasing inflammation. This can be a game-changer for many children because we can identify which foods are aggravating their unique system at the specific time of the testing. (*Not to be confused with food allergies, which cause an immediate reaction.)

Food sensitivity looks at delayed reactions. When you eat something on Monday you don't connect that to how you feel on Wednesday. Therefore, a lot of clients have told me, "Well, that food doesn't make my stomach hurt." They are just not feeling the results until much later. Another key issue is that approximately 80% of kids on the spectrum produce neural antibodies! What does that mean? When kids are eating foods that they are sensitive to, the body can produce antibodies against the cerebellum, the part of the brain that helps you function normally. In short, their body attacks their brain. Food sensitivities don't just affect the gut but also the brain. Many kids with food sensitivities don't have "tummy" issues they have mood, behavior, anxiety, sleep, focus, and sensory issues.

Food sensitivity testing can be done in a variety of ways from drawing blood, saliva, or dried blood spot testing. I prefer the dried blood spot method because it can easily be done from the comfort of your own home.

Comprehensive Organic Acid Testing

Organic acids are chemical compounds that are excreted in the urine of mammals and we humans are mammals! These compounds are created because of the body metabolizing. Metabolism is the act of your body undertaking millions of chemical reactions to help you repair and replenish cells, eliminate waste, and produce energy.

This test can provide a snapshot of overall health and give us an accurate evaluation of yeast, mold, bacteria, and our ability to utilize certain nutrients, neurotransmitter balance, and even how we make energy.

We know that abnormally high levels of metabolic by-products (that's what organic acids are) can cause, or make worse, behavior disorders, hyperactivity, movement disorders, fatigue, and immune function. Organic acid testing is a simple urine test.

Nutrigenomic Testing

This kid-friendly buccal swab test (an oral swab of your cheek cells) can help us predict, with increasing precision, who is more likely to develop specific diseases, who will respond positively or react negatively to a particular drug or supplement therapy, and finally, which nutrients are optimal for a specific individual's health and well-being.

Knowing where the cracks are in our foundation can tell us where we may need the most support. By supporting the cracks with the right diet, nutritional supplements, and lifestyle strategies, you can dramatically increase your child's quality of life.

Nutrigenomics helps to look for typos (called single nucleotide polymorphisms or SNPs) within our genes that predispose us to disease. These SNPs are made by cells that make mistakes when they copy themselves. If you have these SNPs (most of us have them) it does not mean you have or will have a disease. It just means you have a predisposition.

Expose an SNP to the wrong environment, then that gene leans toward disease. Think of this like the Leaning Tower of Pisa. If we use tools to reinforce it, we can slow the tilt in the wrong direction! This kind of testing can then help us to know how to support and provide the body with an optimal environment in which to flourish.

Nutrigenomic testing can serve as a road map to better health and can give us many clues as to why your child experiences certain symptoms. Having knowledge of which way your genes might lean, would tell us where not to put stress.

This is not simply looking at one gene like MTHFR. It is looking at a chain of genes and how our genes are impacted by our diet, lifestyle, and environment. We must look above and beyond one gene to get a clear picture that will help us to create a roadmap to recovery.

Through my years of research and clinical practice, I have created a proprietary genetic panel that is only offered by me and my team. We can correlate 54 specific genes with symptoms your child is experiencing. We go above and beyond MTHFR.

Heavy Metals and Toxic Elements

A simple urine test can help determine if heavy metals and toxic elements have accumulated in the body. Heavy metals, like mercury, can cause heavy metal toxicity which is not easily recognized by conventional medicine or the general public.

Most people have heavy metal accumulation, but they don't know it because symptoms can be vague and mimic other disorders. Heavy metals are used routinely in industrial processes as well as consumer products. Heavy metal toxicity in the body can lead to heavy metal poisoning. and symptoms can include fatigue, migraine headaches, anxiety, depression, poor memory and concentration, learning disorders in children, Parkinson's disease symptoms, or other neurological problems. Toxic heavy metals that commonly accumulate in the human body are mercury (the most toxic heavy metal), lead, cadmium, arsenic, and aluminum.

Toxicants in the environment can also cause underlying problems. A toxicant may act like a hormone (a type of regulatory system), or it may block the production of hormones, block hormone receptors on cells, mimic or amplify the effects of existing hormones or interfere with various bodily functions (such as reproduction, digestion, and respiration). Many toxicants can also cause cancer. Others accumulate in cells or tissues and keep us from producing energy. Yes, toxicants is the right word: a toxin is something found in plants, a toxicant is man-made.

Environmental toxicants can be persistent and hard to break down. They include chemicals such as DDT (an insecticide that has toxic effects on fish, birds, and mammals), polychlorinated biphenyls (PCBs; toxic to fish, other wildlife, and humans), dioxin (a by-product of combustion processes such as chlorine factories or wood pulp mills), and ozone (for example, smog).

There are several ways to test for heavy metals including hair tissue mineral analysis, urine, and stool. Environmental toxicants are also examined using a simple urine test.

Mycotoxins

Mold produces substances called mycotoxins. When mold is allowed to grow on or inside your home it can proliferate and infiltrate your lungs, gut, and skin. As mold spores enter your body, they produce mold metabolites (mycotoxins) that can cause vomiting, nausea, diarrhea, stomach pain and cramps, skin rashes, flu-like symptoms, headaches, fatigue, muscle/joint pain, memory loss, poor circulation, high blood pressure, neurological issues, and even damage to major organs.

Anyone who breathes in mold spores or mold mycotoxins can be affected. That is because the toxins bypass your normal immune system defenses. They can circulate throughout your entire body by attaching themselves to your cells, disrupting functions – all without detection by white blood cells, your protective army.

Not only is it important to test your child for mold toxins but it is also important to test your home if results come back positive. Mycotoxin testing involves a urine sample and can also be detected in an organic acids sample.

Neural Inflammation

A neural inflammation test can determine if you are experiencing inflammation in your brain and spinal cord. Neural inflammation testing can zero in on antigens and autoantibodies associated with a range of neurological disorders. This allows for early detection and therefore prevention of certain neurological issues. Autoantibodies can lead to an attack on one's own body instead of foreign invaders.

This test can be done with serum blood or a dried blood spot.

The body is a complex set of systems, and your child's symptoms are never going to be isolated in one area or system, they are all intertwined!

Therefore, it's so essential to run several tests at once to look at genes, digestion, immunity, detoxification, energy, and neurological function so you can find out why they are or aren't working together. Testing helps us to target healing opportunities so that we can create a clear path and goals.

There are other options besides a pill to help get to the root of your child's health problems.

How Do I Get My Hands on These Tests?

I know you are thinking, "Where do I even start? How do I order these tests? I don't know how to read lab data!"

Many people do not know that anyone can order lab testing, you just need to know where to look. Most of the tests I listed above can be ordered from various labs and you can self-test at home.

Although anyone can order lab testing right off the internet, not all testing is the same. You might be tempted to run down to the drug store and grab one of those genetic tests off the shelf or order a food sensitivity test on Facebook, but those are novelty tests. They are meant for fun and do not provide the crucial data needed to help your child's Tics. Many of those tests are monogenic and look at genes in a way that makes them seem to stand alone in isolation but many genes function in a chain and you need testing that gives you the connection. Plus, who wants to sort through 12,000 pages of raw data?

I have worked with many families who show up with handfuls of test results and no idea what they mean or how to connect the dots. Most have spent thousands of dollars trying to figure it out for themselves but lack the knowledge and expertise to put it all together. If you are hoping to use functional testing to map out your child's Tics, you need to find an expert who knows the right tests to run and what they mean for your child. I promise this will save a lot of time, frustration, and money.

It's not hard to get your hand on the testing, the problem is finding someone who is qualified to interpret the results for you. When I work with clients.

I compare their functional lab data, health history, diet, and current symptoms (Comprehensive Neuro-Immune Analysis). I use all this information to create a step-by-step individualized plan for each person. Many people who run functional lab work may only look at the results on paper, which means they see the results and they tell you everything looks normal. However, sometimes you may exhibit symptoms and there may be hidden clues in your results. It's important to find a provider who knows how to look for those clues and how they apply to your child's specific body.

Chapter 7

Whole Foods

Aside from the genes, lifestyle, and environment, one of the most important factors to consider when looking at your child's Tic symptoms is diet. Diet has a strong relationship with almost every symptom, disease, or health condition as it acts as a catalyst or an inhibitor to the progress of the ailment. In fact, many ailments have been treated through the use of diet control and restrictions. As a result, many people have wondered about the effect of diet on their health, particularly with respect to Tic disorders and their co-diagnoses.

Unfortunately, there has been very limited information and studies in regard to the impact of diet on Tics. It is difficult to get funding for a study on nutrition because most scientific study is provided by big pharma. It's all about the Benjamins!

That leaves us with clinical experience and many parents wonder if there is a dietary solution to all of this. The truth is that food can have tremendous effects on managing the symptoms of Tic disorders. In fact, some people claim that they have been able to manage the symptoms of Tic disorders mainly through their diet.

Furthermore, several studies have shown that there is a strong relationship between your diet and your health, thus further proving the importance of what you eat. Diet and lifestyle improvements are also known to help in reducing Tic symptoms. Diet can also help in coping with syndromes such as ADHD and Autism.

This, then, brings to light an important question on what to eat and what not to eat. There are a lot of opinions as to what to eat to boost your immune system and enhance your health. Ultimately, most people are confused by the array of information at their disposal and are left with more questions than they originally had.

The fact remains that there isn't a clear-cut answer or formula for what is the most appropriate diet. Various body types and compositions require different nutrients to be able to function at their best. However, certain meals can be of great help to parents to help their children cope with the symptoms of

Tic disorders. Many foods help control blood sugar, reduce inflammation, and provide plenty of nutrients.

As a Doctor of Holistic Nutrition, I know the value of a nutrient-dense, whole-food diet, not only in my own family, but also with all of my clients. In the United States, we follow a Standard American Diet (SAD). The SAD is truly sad – it consists of ultra-processed foods in which most of the calories come from carbohydrates and added sugars, as opposed to whole foods that are loaded with fiber and nutrients.

Many of our children are malnourished but their inadequate nutrition isn't from lack of food. Most of them have plenty of food. It is a lack of nutrient-dense food. When we lack the nutrients we need to function, our bodies are left wanting more and children will then tend to eat more junk to fill the void. However, these poor diets can have even more serious ramifications for children with chronic diseases. We are led to believe we need grains, starches, processed snacks, and sweets/desserts. SAD has been linked to increased risk factors that lead to obesity, type 2 diabetes, and unhealthy cholesterol levels, and it most certainly impacts your immune system and inflammation. If you are trying to reduce Tic symptoms, SAD is one you should avoid.

It can take up to six months or longer to see results from a diet change. Some people do see drastic changes within the first couple of weeks but for a lot of people the healing is happening on the inside and that takes time for it to show up on the outside. Parents say, 'We tried a gluten-free diet for two weeks and it didn't help.' Two weeks is not long enough to see positive changes in symptoms. Also, when you make changes to the diet alone, you are not accounting for many of the other imbalances that may be happening in the body. Several foods – gluten being the worst offender – can cause your immune system to make antibodies that can take up to two years to reduce. Keep in mind that dietary changes should be for the long haul.

If you have been following me for a while, you may have seen some of these suggestions before, but they are always worth repeating. My ditch, dump, and dial method are a great place to start for any family.

While there are meals that can help reset the nervous system of the body, there are also meals that aggravate the symptoms of Tics or Tourette's syndrome. Studies have shown that foods such as wheat, milk, eggs, corn, potatoes, beef, chocolate, coffee, citrus, and beans are capable of producing negative neurological reactions that can aggravate those symptoms.

Where should you start when it comes to diet? Here are a few simple steps you can take right now. This is only your starting block but when you include food sensitivity testing, you can refine the diet and create a plan that is based on your unique child.

YOUR DIET CHECK LIST:

Ditch the Junk Food: One important step in approaching Tics is to eliminate many of the unhealthy foods that may be causing underlying inflammation, which impacts the gut and brain. Foods that come from a box or a bag with a barcode are full of sugar, artificial sweeteners, artificial colors, and other nasty additives. These foods are low on nutrients and are not providing your child with what they need to flourish. Eating these foods can lead to a leaky gut, which has an impact on your brain and immune system. Children with Tics are more likely to struggle with inflammation and leaky gut. Studies show that white sugar can also increase Tics.

Refined Sugar: Refined sugars have been known to worsen neurological disorders, such as Tourette's syndrome. Refined sugar causes instability and an increase in the blood sugar level, which leads to hyperactivity, mood swings, and inattention. Sugar intake helps increase dopamine in the brain, thus reducing its production as well as the functions of the receptors. The production of dopamine is vital to managing Tic disorders, as they are connected with the dysfunction in the dopamine system within the brain. Therefore, consuming sugar has a detrimental effect on dopamine levels, which can lead to an increase in Tic symptoms in children.

Parents then have the enormous responsibility of helping their kids refrain from sweets or refined sugar. In fact, sweets and carbonated drinks made of white sugar have been found to worsen Tic symptoms.

Dump the Gluten and Dairy: Foods containing gluten and dairy are inflammatory, which can lead to leaky gut and can also actually act like opioids in the brain. Just like your brain responds to a drug like heroin it responds the same way to gluten and dairy. All of the most addictive foods contain gluten and dairy. Many of them are processed junk as we talked about in step one. Due to their addictive nature, gluten and dairy can impact mood, behavior, and even your child's ability to focus. Several dairy and wheat products also contain higher levels of glutamate, which will excite the brain and may lead to increased Tics. They can also lead to an autoimmune response in the body.

Gluten consumption, celiac disease, and wheat allergies are all associated with neurological conditions. Studies also show that gluten consumption and celiac disease cause an increase in Tics. Recent discoveries have shown that non-celiac gluten sensitivity is also connected to neurological causes. Most of my clients will tell you that taking out gluten makes a big impact.

Many symptoms of non-celiac gluten sensitivity may impact the gastrointestinal tract, but gluten is just as likely, or even more likely, to impact the brain and neurological system. Gluten can harm the brain through inflammation as an excitotoxin (glutamate) and by being broken down during the digestion process into opiate-like peptides like gluteomorphins. It can drastically change brain function and behavior.

Dial in on Nutrition: Just because you have ditched and dumped the junk doesn't mean that everything else is fine. Now is the time to dial in on a nutrient-rich diet. Food is pretty powerful! What your child puts in their mouth will have a direct impact on every cell, tissue, organ, and system in the body. If you think about a water balloon, it's full and nothing else is getting in. When our cells are full of junk the nutrients our kids need to focus and function are not getting in either. You will want to focus on nutritious meats, poultry, eggs, wild-caught fish, fruits, veggies, and even some gluten-free whole grains. You will also want to make sure your child is getting plenty of healthy fats from avocado, nuts, seeds, olive, and coconut oil. Stay away from the foods that come in a box or a bag with a barcode.

Stay Away from Caffeine: Caffeine is a substance that is commonly found in drinks, teas, and coffee. It is used as a stimulant in drugs and medications like Ritalin. Caffeine has been proven to increase Tics so try to keep your children away from caffeine as it can increase their symptoms and episodes.

A note on Nutrient Deficiency

Our children breathe more, eat more, and double in weight and size by the time they are 20 years old. This means that they require more high-quality nutrients to grow. If you have a child who is chronically ill, it is likely that they live in a state of 'fight or flight'. Think back to high school biology when we learned about the saber-tooth tiger chasing us through the forest. If you are out for a walk and a rabid dog shows up, your body is going to immediately have to decide whether to run or fight. This is what happens when our children are constantly struggling with hidden stressors – their bodies end up in a state of constant fight or flight. We know that a body under chronic stress utilizes nutrients at a much faster rate. If your child is growing rapidly and they are in a chronic state of fight or flight, they are going to need far more nutrients than the average child. You also have to take into account genetic status. If we are genetically predisposed to not utilizing certain nutrients that can impact our nutrient deficiency, this is important information we need to know and take into consideration.

Don't be fooled by the letters RDA (Recommended Dietary Allowance). RDA recommendations are the minimal recommendations for nutrients to keep your child from getting sick, designed simply to keep them from getting scurvy and rickets. The RDA is not meant to give your child optimal health, nor does it take into account your child's chronic illness and nutrient deficiency.

Chronically ill children may need significantly more nutrients, period.

NUTRIENT-DENSE FOODS INCLUDE

Avocado or olive oil for cooking and basting: These oils are made up of nutritious essential fatty acids that are necessary to give energy.

Carbohydrates: These are energy-giving foods and can be found in whole food sources like potatoes, beans, and squash. Don't be fooled by the promotion of whole grains! We get far more fiber from fruits and veggies.

Cranberries and blueberries: These are rich in antioxidants that help in repairing damage and boost the immune system of the human body. Ultimately, the body gets all the nutrients it needs as the nervous system is enhanced as well, thereby helping to deal with the symptoms of Tourette's syndrome.

Protein: Proteins are particularly helpful in regulating your sugar level and building up your cells. It is also essential for amino acids, which are the building blocks of our neurotransmitters. Proteins such as wild-caught fish, grass-fed beef, wild game, and pastured poultry.

Water: This is probably one of the most underrated things in a diet, yet it is arguably the most important part of any food. The entire body is made up of at least 60% water, while the brain has more than 70% water. This underlines the importance of water in the human body. Get a filter on your fridge, sink, or whole house to filter out any toxins and chlorine. Clean, pure water is essential for your health.

Organic whole foods: Normally, organic foods are assumed to contain higher nutrients than processed foods that have been subjected to heat, preservatives, and many other processes meant to preserve them. Therefore, non-processed food must be considered to give the body the necessary nutrients in abundance. Eating organic also helps to free you from toxic chemicals sprayed on and around your foods. Check out EWG.org for a list of the dirty dozen and clean 15. These lists will show you the most chemical-laden foods and those that are safer to eat when purchasing non-organic.

A study in 2015 showed that some individuals with Tourette's syndrome eat less than most and are deficient in most of the necessary nutrients, thereby worsening their symptoms. In some other cases, they suffer from nutritional imbalance as they are usually deficient in vitamins and proteins, exposing the body to several threats, including Tic symptoms.

Magnesium- and vitamin B6-rich food: Supplements such as magnesium and vitamin B6 have been shown to help patients gain remarkable improvements in

their symptoms. Research that was published in the *Medicina Clínica* in November 2008 recorded that the presence of vitamins B6 and magnesium have helped improve the symptoms of Tourette's. Therefore, foods such as dark green leafy vegetables, legumes, and grains that are rich in magnesium should be consumed by Tourette's patients. Also, fish, starchy vegetables, organ meats, fortified breakfast cereals, and non-citrus fruits should be encouraged for Tic disorders. Keep in mind that this is an older study and magnesium and B6 are not the only deficiencies your child may be experiencing.

Foods rich in omega-3 fats: In June 2012, pediatric research was published that proved that taking 250 to 500 milligrams of omega-3 fats every day helps in reducing the symptoms and damage experienced by children who have Tourette's syndrome or Tics. Omega-3 fatty acids have also been proven to help enhance the functions of the brain and deal with several neurological issues.

To help your child deal with Tic symptoms, you might want to consider increasing the amount of fish, and walnuts and even adding in an omega-3 supplement. For instance, you could begin with a shrimp that contains at least 267 milligrams of omega-3 fats or a wild Atlantic salmon that contains over 1,500 milligrams of healthy fats. Other examples of foods rich in omega-3 fats are sardines, tuna, flax seeds, walnuts, and grass-fed beef.

Chapter 8

Sugar Detox

We briefly mentioned ditching sugar in Chapter 7 but I truly believe in this day and age we need to address the elephant in the room and her name is sugar!

There are several pieces of evidence that show sugar provides physiological and behavioral effects similar to addictive drugs. In fact, many have asserted that sugar is more addictive than cocaine. Another research study proved that continuous exposure to a high amount of sugar could result in brain changes or adaptation that is similar to nicotine addictions. Animal studies also showed that when sugar is removed from a rat's diet, they show an opiate withdrawal symptom, resulting in anxious behavior and a reduction in the release of dopamine. Sugar is a luxury that young children suffering from Tourette's syndrome cannot afford. Dopamine helps reward and control pleasure, which can affect the symptoms of Tics or Tourette's syndrome.

Sugar detox is essential for anyone who intends to take their health seriously. Despite the immense benefits that sugar detox has, it still comes with its downside that must be properly managed. In a bid to avoid the many ills and disadvantages of sugar intake, such as weight gain, diabetes, and fatigue, many have cut off sugar very abruptly from their diet.

It is important to safely remove sugar, which is an integral part of anyone's nutrient intake, slowly from your diet. For most people, the symptoms are mild and temporary; however, the sudden loss of sugar in children and young teenagers with Tics and Tourette's disorder might cause their conditions to worsen temporarily. These symptoms may include an increased craving for high-calorie foods, lack of energy, muscle aches, bloating, stomach cramps, irritability, depression, and nausea.

Your Turn: How to Safely Sugar Detox

Fiber is a must-have when dealing with symptoms of sugar detox. It can help us deal with cravings and also help in regulating the sugar levels in the body. Magnesium-rich foods are also a great help to support fluctuating blood sugar levels. These include beef, poultry, pumpkin seeds, almonds, and black beans.

Knowing full well that sugar is extremely addictive, how can you help your child break free from their addiction and reduce the craving? Here are some tips to help you achieve this:

1. Consume protein products to curb the appetite.
2. Drink enough water to allow for optimum hydration.
3. Exercise frequently to enhance the release of endorphins to regulate blood sugar levels.
4. Eat more fresh fruits and veggies which will provide a nice boost of fiber.
5. Get enough rest and sleep. According to a study in 2018, lack of sleep can result in cravings for bad foods.
6. Learn to relax and deal with stress.

Chapter 9

Gut Health

The gut is an integral part of the human body as it is connected to most of the other bodily systems. Research carried out for more than two decades, proves the importance of the gut system and its relationship with the immune system, mental health, mood, autoimmune diseases, skin disorders, endocrine issues, cancer, and other diseases. The gut system used to not be seen as a complex system, but rather as a long tube that food goes through, is absorbed in, and later excreted. However, the human digestive system is much more than that. Our guts include an entire universe of bacteria that makes up the microbiome, microorganisms that live in our intestines. The human digestive system has at least 300 to 500 species of bacteria, which all play an important role in the entire system's health. To be honest, you have more bacterial cells in your body than human cells. You are more bacteria than human!

The gut's health affects the entire body, which is particularly true in people suffering from Tics or Tourette's syndrome, as it most harshly affects the neurological system and the mood. Dr. Eamonn Quigley stated in his *Journal of Gastroenterology and Hepatology* that having a wide range of bacteria can help support the immune system, depression, obesity, and other conditions that can aggravate Tourette's conditions. In short, having an unhealthy gut can lead to the aggravation of Tourette's syndrome or Tics symptoms.

How to Identify an Unhealthy Gut

Your child may have a Tic but we know that these symptoms are not purely neurological. Many children also experience chronic stomach aches, gas, bloating, mood swings, or trouble sleeping. These symptoms can all stem from the gut and are signs that it is time to find out more.

Tics result when activity in certain parts of the brain become unregulated leading to excessive movement or vocalization. Tic disorders have many different causes – including genetics, trauma, and infection – but they share common symptoms, such as eye blinking, grimacing of the face, uncontrollable movements and vocal noises.

Put simply, the gut and the brain are connected. This connection can have an impact on your child's Tics. Let's start with the Vagus nerve that connects the gut and brain. It controls the release of hormones, including serotonin, which reduces inflammation and is essential for healthy gut function. Toxicity in the body can damage this nerve, which can impact brain function and increase Tics. Toxins that are released by harmful bacteria such as yeast, fungus and parasites can contribute to inflammation that can degrade the Vagus nerve. Toxins from medications, artificial sweeteners, and food additives also contribute to this problem.

Gut health includes the health of your microbiome (gut flora or gut bugs), which controls several bodily functions, including digestion, immunity, and central nervous system function (including Tic disorders). Information from thousands of studies shows how important it is to support healthy gut microbiota (gut bugs) to improve immune, neurological and digestive issues for children with Tics.

Some of the additional symptoms of poor gut health include ADHD, OCD, mood disorders, meltdowns or sensory issues. As I mentioned earlier, sleep issues, stomach aches, constipation, diarrhea, rashes, hives, and other skin issues can also point to problems in the gut. It can also take a lot of personal energy to cope with pervasive Tic symptoms and the feeling that one cannot control them. This can actually cause our children to use more nutrients leading to nutrient deficiency. If your child already has gut problems, they may not be absorbing enough nutrients in the first place.

YOUR TURN: IS YOUR CHILD'S GUT A HOT MESS?

Upset stomach and poopy pants: Bloating, diarrhea, heartburn, gas, and constipation are indications of an unhealthy gut. A healthy gut will have no problems processing food and excreting waste. Constipation and loose stools are common gut problems. A note on constipation, you should be going #2 at least once a day. If you are going a day or two without a poo, you are constipated. Constipation occurs as a result of changes in diet, medication, being less active, and illness. Loose stools, on the other hand, are bowel movements that are abnormally watery. They often occur after eating. Causes of loose stools include certain foods, food poisoning, or IBS.

A high concentration of sugar in your diet: A high concentration of sugar or sweetener in your meals reduces the number of bacteria and microbiota within the gut, thus reducing its health. This anomaly will also increase the number of bacteria within the gut and affect the entire system further. An increase in the amount of sugar through a high fructose syrup leads to inflammation.

Sudden weight changes: Gaining unnecessary weight without any alteration in your diet can be a sign that you have an unhealthy gut. The imbalance in the gut often leads to an impaired gut, which affects the ability of the body to absorb nutrients, store fat and maintain blood sugar. Weight loss is often affected by small intestine bacterial overgrowth (SIBO), while weight gain is a consequence of the resistance to insulin and the increased urge of overeating due to the failure of absorption.

Autoimmune conditions: Medical researchers have discovered that the gut system is responsible for inflammation that can result in autoimmune conditions. Autoimmune disease is a condition that allows the body to attack the antibodies instead of the harmful agents of the body.

Skin irritation: Eczema is a sign that the gut has been damaged. Skin irritation occurs mostly due to allergies which are caused by a protein deficiency resulting in leaking of the gut.

Sleep disturbances or constant fatigue: An unhealthy gut leads to bad sleep and insomnia, which causes fatigue. The hormone that causes rest, serotonin, is produced within the gut. An imbalance in the gut can lead to insomnia.

Food intolerances: Food intolerances are often a sign of an unhealthy gut. Symptoms such as bloating, fatigue, diarrhea, rashes, acid reflux, and nausea are often associated with your digestive health. Therefore, being able to discover the foods that trigger those symptoms will do your health a world of good and help boost your digestive system.

Bad moods: By now you know that the gut and the brain are connected, and the gut microbiota influences that interaction. They also play an important role in regulating what is absorbed by the body and what is excreted. If your child is experiencing mood swings and meltdowns, it's time to look at the gut.

Tics, ADHD, SPD, OCD, Dysgraphia, Dyslexia, brain fog, anxiety: Check, check, and double-check. If your child is experiencing more than two of the symptoms listed in this section it's time to look to the gut.

WHAT TO DO ABOUT AN UNHEALTHY GUT

Since the gut is also referred to as the digestive system, food and waste are the only things that pass through there. So how then can the system be treated through food and help a child suffering from Tics or Tourette's syndrome? Here are a group of foods that can be used to treat an unhealthy gut:

- Foods rich in fiber: Foods that are rich in fiber or have high fiber concentration like beans, legumes, bananas, asparagus, berries, leeks, and oats have been proven to have tremendous health benefits on the gut.
- Fermented foods: Foods such as sauerkraut, yogurt, tempeh, miso, and kefir are fermented foods that are excellent sources of dietary protein. These dietary proteins help enhance the growth and presence of gut microbiota that enhance the overall health of the gut. Although the quality of the food may vary, the effect of the food is there, nonetheless.
- Garlic and onion: Much more than the anti-cancer and immune system enhancing properties they possess, onions and garlic have properties that help boost the gut system.
- Collagen-boosting foods: Bone broth at meals has been proven to be extremely helpful in helping seal the gut lining, as it is extremely rich in collagen. To get the most out of your diet you can also try collagen-rich foods such as meats, mushrooms, salmon and eggs.

Get Enough Rest and Sleep

Gut health affects the brain, immune system, neurological health system, and the entire body. Therefore, to enhance the health of your gut and see its effects on the occurrence of Tic disorders, it is vital that you change some of your lifestyle and habits. An important aspect of your habits or lifestyle is rest, as it also helps to improve the health of the gut.

Chapter 10

Toxins in Your Home

The advent of technology has changed the world as a whole. In the quest to find ways to make life easier, we might have made it more dangerous through the presence of toxicants. Scientifically, toxicants are a toxic substance. Toxins are harmful substances produced within living cells or organisms. Some hard-core science people will rip my head off here, but for the purpose of this book and how society addresses toxicants, we are going to call them toxins.

Unfortunately, toxins have become a part of our daily lives. People are unaware of the excessive amount of toxins that they are using in and around their homes, schools, offices, gyms, farms, fields, and lives. In fact, most of the materials used in the building industry are found all over the world and are not without their consequences or demerits. Several problems have arisen, such as immune system disorder, fatigue disorder, hormonal imbalance, nausea, and neurological disorder.

All of these symptoms can aggravate several neurological conditions, such as Tic disorders and Tourette's syndrome. A report by *The British Medical Journal* in 2004 stated that the environment and lifestyle of individuals are the major determinants of diseases. A study also revealed that most Americans have at least 400 to 800 chemicals stored within the fat cells of their bodies. Therefore, for you to effectively manage Tics and nurse your child back to health, you need to focus not only on the lifestyle of your child through food and diet but also on the environment of your child through the management of toxins.

Every time this aspect of Tic management comes up, people tend to get surprised and wonder how they can possibly control toxin overload. They always believe that toxins come from the outside and that there is little or nothing that can be done to control them. This is far from the truth. In fact, a study shows that there is a higher concentration of toxins present within the home compared to that outside. How is this so? In a bid to get the best in aesthetics and comfort, people have made use of technology as well as different substances that generate a lot of toxins within an enclosed space.

How then can any parent make the home free of harmful toxins which can serve as triggers or aggravate Tourette's syndrome? Although it is almost impossible to know all the toxins in the material used in building your house, there are a few steps that you can take to make your job less herculean:

- Be aware of all the major toxins common within homes
- Know the safe substitutes to replace them with or reduce the danger they pose
- Find out if you can do without those products permanently
- Always try to ventilate your home to reduce the concentration of such toxins within the home and release them to produce cleaner air
- Plant flowers or plants in pots and vases, as plants help trap harmful toxins

COMMON TOXINS IN THE HOME AND WHERE TO LOOK FOR THEM

Toxins are all around us and within our homes. This is a source of concern for people who are trying to lead a healthy life, as it interferes with their health and productivity. As a result, many people have always sought to get rid of toxins, particularly within the home. No surprise really, as the home has been proven to contain a higher concentration of toxins than outside. Furthermore, getting rid of the toxins outside is not feasible, as you can't deal with all the sources as an individual. Therefore, most people are concerned with getting rid of the toxins within the home, an area they can largely control.

Despite the home being an enclosed space, it is still a herculean task to hope to eliminate the toxins without knowing them. Here are some of the toxins that are common within our air, food, and water:

VOLATILE ORGANIC COMPOUNDS (VOCS)

Volatile Organic Compounds are chemical compounds that vaporize easily and exist in the form of vapor gas pollutants. VOCs are very common within most households with at least 200 being present in carpets. The EPA stated that VOCs are more present within the home, not because of the enclosed space, but due to the household materials within.

Health Hazards and Threats: The compound is known to cause headaches, visual disorders, memory loss, and dizziness which might aggravate the symptoms of Tourette's syndrome. People with respiratory diseases are prone to illness and irritations as a result of the compound. Furthermore, consistent exposure often results in liver and kidney damage, cancer, and the impairment of the central nervous system, which is critical to Tourette's syndrome.

Sources: VOCs are found in materials such as carpets, interior paints, particle boards, plywood and pressed wood products, new plastics, electronics, shampoos, deodorants, cleaning fluids, moth repellants, stoves and tobacco products.

How to Reduce Exposure

- Don't use products with a high VOC content: Always try to buy low-VOC and zero-VOC paints to use in your house. You should also try to buy solid wood, plywood, and hardboard instead of pressed wood. It is also important that you discourage smoking in all forms within your home.

- Air dry new products outside: It is essential that you allow fresh ventilat-ion anytime you buy a new carpet, linoleum, or have used paints. Open the doors and windows and turn on the fans if possible.

- Regulate the Temperature of the Room: You could also attempt to maintain the temperature of the room and keep it low. When your home's temperature is kept low, you will be able to reduce the amount of gas emission from substances such as VOCs and formaldehyde from being infused into your environment.

PESTICIDES

The EPA recorded that about 60% of herbicides, 90% of pesticides, and 30% of insecticides have cancerous properties. Unfortunately, at least 50% to 95% of foods in the United States contain residue of pesticides.

Threats: Pesticides are harmful substances that pose great danger to the eyes and throat and may result in cancer. It also poses a threat to the nervous system as it affects young patients suffering from Tourette's syndrome and Tics.

Sources: Foods contain a large number of pesticides. Other household danger zones are sprays, and lawns having been treated with insecticides and pesticides which then stray indoors.

How to Reduce Exposure:

- Begin a "No shoe policy" within your home: One of the easiest ways to keep pesticides out of the home is to ask that people take their shoes off and leave them outside before entering your home. While it might seem old-fashioned, its advantages are still of immense benefit. You could give visitors or friends cheap shoes to wear if they are uncomfortable with taking off their shoes. Doing this will ensure that pesticides will not be trapped in shoes and brought into the home to aggravate the conditions of Tourette's syndrome patients.

- Always try to use fresh organic fruits: It is often difficult to stick to anything that is fresh and organic, as most fruits barely are. The best way to remedy this is to try to get healthy fruits on your own by planting a backyard garden. You could also select foods or fruits that have been proven to have a low concentration of pesticides. You could also choose to buy fresh, organically bred eggs from free-range birds, as they are free from toxins.

- Utilize natural pest control means: A natural lawn will help deal with pests and weeds, restraining them without pesticides. A more natural means of controlling pests, such as the use of diatomaceous earth, kills insects or pests naturally. You should be able to control harmful pests and substances naturally without the help of a pesticide. Ultimately, pesticides should be used only as a last resort when other remedies and pest control measures have failed.

FUNGAL TOXINS

Allergies are triggers that patients who have Tics or Tourette's syndrome always try to avoid as they always create stress and anxiety. Unfortunately, allergic reactions to mold are quite common - at least one in three people is allergic to mold. Even in small amounts, fungal toxins, also known as mycotoxins, could result in many health problems.

Health Hazards and Threats: Scientists have not discovered any definite evidence of the health hazards and threats posed by mycotoxins. However, there are several toxic effects established already which can serve as Tic triggers, such as suppression of the immune system, irritation of the mucus membrane, and the impairment of the nervous system.

Sources: Molds, fungal toxins, or mycotoxins can be found in wet areas with regular temperature changes, air-conditioning units, and buildings.

How to Reduce Exposure:

- Try to maintain cleanliness on filters through heating, air-conditioning, and ventilating systems.
- Always try to keep a dry environment by drying out the moisture and getting rid of water sources around the area of the mold.

- Always maintain a humidity of less than 60%. To achieve this, you may need a dehumidifier in some areas.
- Keep items with a high concentration of cellulose in dry environments.

PHTHALATES AND PVC (POLYVINYL CHLORIDE)

Polyvinyl Chloride (PVC) is a chemical compound made up of phthalates that is used by many industries. It is also referred to as alkyl aryl esters or dialkyl of carboxylic esters. There are several phthalates with diverse uses as well as different toxic properties. PVCs are mostly used in softening hard plastics and in increasing the life of fragrances.

Health Hazards and Threats: PVCs have been discovered to affect children's health through the endocrine system. Consistent exposure to PVCs is particularly dangerous to children and anyone suffering from Tourette's syndrome or Tics as it affects their hormones. The PVCs try to mimic the hormones' chemical features and properties. Furthermore, pregnant women are also at risk as it affects the embryonic development of the genitals of the child. Unfortunately, these risks are still prevalent even in exposures of minute quantities.

Sources: PVCs are present in plastic bottles, food storage containers, and other food containers, indirectly passing phthalates into food. PVCs are also present in consumer products such as drapes, wall coverings, babies' toys, curtains, cosmetics, vinyl flooring, and fixatives.

How to Reduce Exposure:

- You must check your child's toys for PVCs or phthalates before buying them.
- Anytime you are buying plastic materials, you must ask if they contain phthalates.
- Do not eat food kept or microwaved in PVC plastics.
- You can look out for recycling code #3 to identify PVC products before buying them.
- Try to always buy PVC-free draperies, shades, and curtains. To achieve success, you could buy more natural fiber materials such as cotton, wool, hemp, silk, and bamboo.
- Always ensure that your house is well-ventilated to flush out the toxins.

DIOXINS

Dioxins are produced through the incomplete combustion of commercial or municipal waste, such as chlorine bleaching of paper, incineration, and burning of wood, oil, and other forms of fuels.

Health Hazards and Threats: Dioxins can lead to cancer, skin discoloration, chlorate, skin rashes, and mild liver damage.

Sources: Most of the exposure to dioxins comes from consuming commercial animal fats. At least more than 20% of exposure to dioxins comes from milk and dairy products. The bulk of the exposure comes from beef, fish, eggs, and poultry. Toxins in fish accumulate, making the toxic levels extremely high (as much as 100,000 times the amount of toxins in the environment). Dioxins are also found in cigarettes, although the portion is in very small quantities. There are also small traces of dioxins within the atmosphere.

How to Reduce Exposure:

- Eat organic grass-fed, pastured, and wild caught.
- Cut your consumption of non-organic meat and dairy products.
- Do not burn substances that contain chlorine, such as plastic and wood.

These also have PCP on them.

HEAVY METALS

Metals such as lead, mercury, aluminum, and cadmium, because they are heavier in weight, can make them dominant in our environment and be stored up in soft tissues in the body.

Health Hazards and Threats: Heavy metals have been the cause of neurological disorders, foggy head, nausea, fatigue, low production of red and white blood cells, abnormal heart rhythms, cancer, and Alzheimer's.

Sources: Heavy metals can be found in drinking water, vaccines, pesticides, antiperspirants, dental amalgams, chlorine plants, building materials, and lead paints.

How to Reduce Exposure:

- Use water filters.

- Always use cold water for drinking, cooking, or for making coffee and tea.
- You should also not eat fish known to contain high levels of mercury, such as king mackerel, swordfish, orange roughy, tilefish, and marlin. You should also try to set a limit on the amount of tuna consumed, canned 'white' albacore, and steak.
- Check to see if your home was built in the 1970s, as the paints used in that period were largely lead-based.
- Do not buy products that are made with PFC, such as Scotchgard and Teflon cookware.
- Do not use treated wood such as ACZA or CCA on your children's wooden toys, tree houses, or any wooden structure for children.

POLYBROMINATED DIPHENYL ETHERS (PBDES)

PBDEs are toxic chemicals that have been used as flame retardants in big industries for more than 30 years. Although PBDEs are no longer prevalent or as commonly used as before, they are still used in North America.

Health Hazards and Threats: Recent research carried out on laboratory animals has connected the exposure of PBDEs to a series of health hazards. Examples of such health situations are thyroid hormone disruption, hearing deficits, delayed puberty onset, decreased sperm count, cancer, permanent learning, memory impairment, and fetal malformation.

Sources: PBDEs can be found in furniture, furniture cushions, mattresses, pet beds, household electronics and appliances, and carpet and carpet paddings.

How to Reduce Exposure:

- Don't let children wear flame-retardant clothing and sleepwear.
- Always choose natural furnishing and bedding. For instance, you should choose wool and cotton over foam and polyester products.
- Eat more fruits and vegetables and cut the number of animal fats you consume.
- Reduce the amount of dust in your environment by damp cleaning.

CHLOROFORM

Chloroform is a colorless liquid that has a nice, slightly sweet, and non-irritating odor. As a result of its appealing smell, it is used in making other chemicals.

Health Hazards and Threats: Chloroform is a compound that is produced when chlorine is added to water and thus infiltrates our environment through our water treatment plants. The treatment of the water rids it of impurities and organic matter, making it safe for drinking and cooking. Chloroform is therefore present in the water and contaminates our food and drinking water.

How to Reduce Exposure:

- Set up a showerhead to keep the temperature of your bathing or shower water low.
- Open the window or use the fan when using hot water for cleaning or taking a shower.
- Put the washer in an area that encourages ventilation, such as the garage.

TIPS TO REDUCE TOXIN LEVELS WITHIN THE HOME

The atmosphere is filled with quite a number of toxins, making it difficult to be able to determine a specific method to deal with them all. The characteristics of these compounds are wide. However, there are several ways through which the level of toxins in the home can be reduced. Here are some of the simplest ones you can do immediately:

Make Use of Natural Cleaning Products in Your Home: Look out for natural cleaning products to be used in your home. In the same vein, you could source ingredients and make your own cleaning products.

Discourage Bringing Shoes into Your Home: Pesticides, herbicides, and other toxins are usually trapped on and brought into the home through shoes. You must encourage the “No shoe” policy in your home. This can be done by asking family members, guests, and friends to take off their shoes at the door before entering your house. Toxins and chemicals have a long half-life and mostly last for several years before their effects wear off.

Refrain from Using Chemical Pest Control: Chemical pest control methods are mostly made up of toxins meant for harmful pests. Unfortunately, these chemicals harm not only the pests but also humans, particularly those suffering from Tics. Several alternatives are safe and without any toxin-related side effects on the health of people. These alternatives are effective in the control of insects and other pests.

Plant Toxin-Reducing Plants: Several researchers have observed that certain plants can trap toxin-containing gases from the atmosphere. These plants have been proven to be highly effective in cleaning up the atmosphere and getting the air within the home clean.

Clean Your Furnace and Ventilating System or Air-conditioning Systems: You must clean your ventilating or air-conditioning systems at least once every three months, depending on how often you use them.

Make Use of Natural Toiletries for Your Child: At first, when I started using natural health and beauty products for Whit, it was an arduous task for me, as it would be for anyone trying out something new. It is easier to walk into any store and just choose toiletries at random. However, being deliberate has always had its advantages, and this is one of them. Choosing natural toiletries has been shown to reduce the number of toxins you are likely to contact. Stop using shampoos, toothpaste, cosmetics, and antiperspirants that are not natural brands or sourced from natural ingredients. Again EWG.org has a page called Skin Deep® that provides great resources for toxin-free toiletries and beauty products.

Stop Using Synthetic Fragrances: Avoid using materials such as artificial air fresheners, fabric softeners, synthetic fragrances, or dryer sheets. These materials are capable of polluting the atmosphere with toxins that are usually inhaled.

Refrain from Using Lawn-Care Chemicals: It is also essential that you stop using chemicals to grow and care for your lawn. Most times, the residues of these chemicals can be trapped in shoes and brought into the home. These residues last for a long period of time. It is better to use natural materials to care for the lawn instead of herbicides, fertilizers, and pesticides.

Get Your Tap Water Tested: These toxins are present in drinking water, especially in the form of chloroform. Therefore, the best way to tackle this is to install a filter and a faucet in your showers and bath.

Make Room for Ventilation: Most new buildings and structures are constructed to be airtight. This implies that there is little or no ventilation in the room, and everywhere is airtight. It is important to aerate your room to allow fresh air and to get rid of harmful toxins.

Here are a few of my favorite resources for finding toxin-free products:

- http://mamaforhealth.com/master-list
- http://www.ewg.org/foodnews/dirty-dozen.php
- http://www.ewg.org/foodnews/clean-fifteen.php
- http://www.ewg.org/skindeep

Chapter 11

Developing Healthy Habits to Cope with Tic Symptoms (What You Need to Change)

Indeed, health is one of the most underrated gifts in life. Rest, exercise and a good diet are prerequisites for developing and maintaining a healthy lifestyle, which is key to helping you and your family cope with Tic symptoms.

Like all health conditions, Tic disorders and other related symptoms can be reduced and even resolved. Your lifestyle and the healthy habits you choose play a crucial role in achieving this. To effectively manage Tic disorders, major lifestyle changes are needed to help your child manage the situation effectively. Alterations in diet, exercise, stress management, and rest will help your child manage their symptoms effectively.

It is important to learn some health tips on dealing with Tics and how they can be incorporated into your lifestyle and the daily routine of your child.

LIFESTYLE TIPS RECOMMENDED WHEN DEALING WITH TICS

Stress

How do you deal with stress in kids with Tics?

As I have previously said, stress is not simply a mental/emotional occurrence. You must consider environmental, biological, and physical stressors as well. In short, this book encompasses the many forms of stress and how they are impacting your child.

It is quite easy to associate stress with adults and think it is a concept that will be foreign to children. The truth is that children experience and are affected by it as much as adults are. Tics and Tourette's syndrome are one of the many consequences of continual stress in children. Reducing the amount of stress that your child experiences can greatly help you in managing their Tics.

Here are some helpful tips you can use to reduce stress for your child:

Engage Your Child: While it might seem weird having your child participate in more activities when they are tired, it is one way to get the best from them and help them deal with stress. Exercise can positively engage your child and get them active. It won't make the stress disappear, but it is an important step in dealing with emotional stress and calming them down and is also great for detoxification. Our lymphatic system does not work on a pump so the only way to move toxins out of our body is to move.

Take Control: There is nothing quite as powerful as an organized life: think schedules, timetables, and routines. This might be boring for those who might want to opt for something more spontaneous. However, the best results are acquired through consistent and deliberate actions which means you need to take charge of your child's activities. You could create a timetable that will keep them entertained and engaged while conserving their energy and reducing stress. This will also help reduce their screen time by keeping them away from the TV or mobile phone for periods of time (especially before bed). You can have some downtime while directing their activities and helping them make the most of their day while they avoid stress.

Encourage Them to Play and Interact with Others: Humans are social beings and connecting is part of our very essence. Socializing with others is not only a form of emotional therapy but also necessary when dealing with stress. Children must relate with their friends, talk, and develop interpersonal skills to help cope with stress. Those who have Tics must be encouraged to interact and connect with their peers to deal with stress and help lift their emotional well-being. It will also help them deal with stigmatism or bullying and other forms of stress.

Encourage Your Kids to Have Personal Time: It is easy for people to become absorbed in work and get carried away by the dividends such work will bring. As parents, we expect the most from our children and tend to push them to their limits and beyond. While we plan their day and schedule their activities, we tend to put in many productive activities, making it difficult for them to have personal time for themselves. We must carve out time to recreate, meditate and be alone, helping them rest and stay away from stress. Teach your kids the tools they need for self-care. As adults, we are the worst at taking care of ourselves and I can't say that anyone ever taught me what self-care was. It is import-ant for your children to understand that to stay healthy and eliminate symptoms that taking care of themselves is important.

Help Them Learn Something New: Learning something new might be challenging, but if the subject is well crafted, children and young people relish such opportunities. Learning helps them explore and opens them up to a new world of possibilities that help them recreate and have fun. For instance, you could teach your child how to swim or teach them how to play the piano, which is calm and engaging. This creates a new world that kids love to explore and helps them cope better with stress.

Teach Them Healthy Habits: This will help them cope with stress and lead a productive life. Discipline is one such habit. Children who are disciplined and know when to stop eating a meal when they have had enough or when to turn the TV off because it is time for bed will be able to lead a more stress-free life when they go to school the following morning. This is an invaluable skill when dealing with Tics.

Being Kind: Research has shown that people who help others are usually more resilient and emotionally healthier. The more they give, the happier they become. Teaching children to be helpful makes them resilient and emotionally stable; hence they become healthy humans and can better cope with stress and Tourette's syndrome.

Teach Them to Work Smart and Not Hard: The world is gradually changing, and it belongs to those who are smart and are willing to show it in their work. Stress is often caused by having to do a lot in such little time which triggers so much anxiety. It is important to teach your child how to work smart and get the most from their efforts. For instance, you could teach your child how to start with the toughest tasks and finish off with the easier ones or start with the most important tasks and prioritize them.

Teach Your Child to Be Positive and Worry Less: Pessimism always brings a lot of worry and worry has never achieved anything. Most times, people who worry are usually stressed out and have a lot of pressure on them. It is the same for young people, as they are stressed and easily discouraged when worried and get to do less in the end. Patients suffering from Tourette's syndrome cannot afford to be worried, as they need to deal with other stressors.

HOW TO DEAL WITH ANXIETY

Sometimes stress can lead to feelings of anxiety. Most of the clients I work with have some level of anxiety added to their list of diagnoses.

Anxiety is another trigger that must be managed if you intend to help your child deal with their Tics. Adults also suffer from anxiety or anxiousness.

Anxiety can trigger Tics and Tics can trigger anxiety; therefore, part of the process involves managing anxiety to effectively manage the stress that comes with it.

However, before a condition can be addressed, its symptoms must be identified. How then can you identify the symptoms?

Symptoms of Anxiety

- Physical Symptoms
- Fast and irregular heartbeat
- Feeling lightheaded and dizzy
- Headache
- Loss of appetite and sweating
- Breathlessness
- Shaking

Mental Symptoms

- Being unable to relax
- Fear
- Inability to sleep and concentrate

Symptoms of Anxiety Specific to Children:

Symptoms can occur at different age groups and at different stages. Some of the symptoms in little children are:

- Irritability, crying, and being clingy
- Being awake at night
- Sleeping difficulty
- Bad dreams
- Bedwetting
- Tummy aches
- Headaches
- Expressing fear
- Panic

Symptoms of Anxiety Observed in Older Children:

- Difficulty in concentrating
- Having issues sleeping or eating
- Pessimism and thinking a lot about bad things happening

- Frequent outbursts
- Avoiding daily activities
- A low level of confidence to try out new things or face daily activities

Causes of Fear or Anxiety

Fear and anxiety are common for everyone to experience. Any time you're feeling anxious or tired, the body releases hormones such as adrenaline and cortisol, which can be quite helpful when you're faced with certain situations or in an emergency. Nevertheless, the constant release of these hormones is not healthy and can exacerbate conditions such as Tics or Tourette's syndrome in children. Your child is in a constant state of "fight or flight" which triggers this constant release of adrenaline and cortisol.

One of the best ways to reduce anxiety is to know its causes and then eliminate them as best you can.

Inflammation, nutritional deficiencies, underlying infections, toxins, and food sensitivities can also contribute to the anxiety your child is experiencing. I was a very anxious child, very fearful, full of panic, scared of the world, and always had a sense of impending doom. I also thought that was all part of my personality. It wasn't until I was in my 30's and straightened out my own health that I discovered that the lifelong anxiety I experienced was not just anxiety but inflammation, nutritional deficiencies, underlying infections, toxins, and food sensitivities as the contributing factors.

Although children get anxious for different reasons and at different stages, many of the sources of worry are seen as "normal" experiences. For instance, children between six months to three years have anxiety with separation from their parents. Often, they become clingy and cry when they are separated from their parents or caregivers.

Children at preschool age develop fears or phobias of certain things or situations. Some of them are afraid of the dark; others are afraid of heights, insects, water, blood, storms, and other animals. However, these phobias tend to go away on their own.

However, as parents, we must always ask, "Why? What are the contributing factors and catalysts that may be driving anxiety?"

As your child grows, the reason for fear changes with the challenges they face at different stages of their life. For example, at some point in the child's life, they might be afraid of a new school, tests, or exams.

Your Turn

How to Help Your Child Deal with Anxiety:

- Always try to converse with a family member, counselor, or health professional.
- Teach your child to use calming techniques to regulate his or her breathing. Deep belly breathing or box breathing are easy techniques that even little ones can do.
- Teach your child how to exercise by running, swimming, and doing yoga, which will help your child relax.
- Help your child sleep as and when due: you could set up a timetable to help them stick to a sleep schedule. If sleeping is difficult, you must find out why sleeping is difficult and help them become better.
- You should always prepare a regular and healthy diet for your child to keep them stable. A healthy diet regulates your child's energy level, their blood sugar level and provides essential nutrients needed for them to thrive.
- Encourage your child to interact with others as talking to others often helps a great deal when you are anxious. Therefore, you must try to teach your child to share their experiences with you or their friends to help calm them down and manage their anxiety.
- Find a group or community that can help the child relax.

How to Help Your Child Deal with Anxiety (the Things Not to Do):

While there are many things to do to help your child deal with anxiety (a trigger for Tics and Tourette's syndrome), there are countless other things that should *not* be done to prevent anxiety in a child. Some such things are:

DON'T Train Your Child to Try to Do Everything at Once: It is important that you set realistic targets for your child and small milestones before they achieve their target. This will take pressure off them and reduce anxiety while increasing their self-confidence and building their self-esteem. This way, they will better be able to deal with Tics and Tourette's syndrome through a reduction in their anxiety levels.

DO Teach Your Child to Stop Spending Energy on Things That They Cannot Change: Every parent needs to teach their children resilience and perseverance. However, there is a thin line between resilience and doing the same thing again and again with no change which often creates stress and unnecessary anxiety. Therefore, you must teach your child to move on and not waste energy on what they cannot change.

Don't Ignore Your Child in Their Moments of Anxiety: It is vital to let your child know that they are not alone when it comes to anxiety and that it is a common thing. You should speak to them in moments of anxiety by creating a safe space for them to share and be listened to.

Don't Avoid Looking Under the Hood: Remember anxiety can be caused by underlying factors like nutrient deficiencies, inflammation, stress, underlying infections, and poor gut health. By utilizing functional lab testing we can start to dig deeper and improve, often even remove, most anxiety symptoms.

Chapter 12

Overtired, Exhausted, And Meltdown City

A child with a Tic disorder and an accompanying long list of symptoms is a child who is in a constant state of fight or flight. Their bodies are on high alert and the red check engine light is going bonkers. They are consistently overtired, over-exhausted, and one step away from meltdown city.

One of the best ways to keep your child from being tired or exhausted is to ensure that they get enough sleep. How can you help a child get to sleep and harness the rest they so need? How can a child be made to relax and helped to sleep the way they ought to? Here are some tips to help you achieve this:

A Warm Bath: A warm bath will help calm a child's nerves and prepare them for sleep.

Dim the Lights: You must dim the light for your child to sleep effectively. Lowering the lights helps encourage the body to sleep as it encourages the production of melatonin, a sleep hormone.

Help Your Child Read or Listen to Some Soothing Music to Calm Their Nerves: You could encourage your child to read silently or listen to a piece of relaxing music that helps to create a relaxed environment. You could also help guide your child through some breathing exercises to relax before going to bed.

Avoid Screens in Your Child's Room: No kid wants to turn off their favorite cartoon or TV show when they know they are going to school the next day. It is difficult to expect children to show restraint or self-control the same way adults are expected to. Tablets, laptops, and television can affect the sleep of children. It is important that you keep children's screens away from them and have them charge them in another room. You should also ensure that your child stops using their gadgets at least an hour before sleep time.

The Structure of Your Child's Bedroom: Dark rooms help to create an optimal sleep environment. A moderately dark and clean room helps your child relax and sleep effectively. You should also ensure that the room is properly ventilated and kept at about 16 to 20 degrees Celsius. You could also fit some dark curtains to block light and filter roof noise. If you're living in a noisy environment, you could get some double glazing done or get some earplugs for your child.

Feeding Enough to Deal with Fatigue: One of the best ways to keep energy levels up is to eat properly. You might have to introduce healthy snacks and fruits into your child's diet to eat every three to four hours to keep their energy levels up.

Exercise: Most times, when you're tired, exercise is the last thing on your mind; however, from a clinical perspective, exercise can improve sleep.

Proper Sleep: Proper sleep prevents the body from getting tired easily. Sleep remains one of the best ways to recharge and stay alert throughout the day. Most people get carried away with their activities; they are engrossed and sacrifice time for sleep instead. However, the role of sleep cannot be ignored. It is important to encourage good sleeping habits by taking them to bed early and waking up early. You should also help them avoid taking naps during the day and encourage them to rest before going to bed. This will give them enough time to rest, avoid being tired and prevent Tics from occurring.

If you are still finding it difficult to help your child sleep after these processes, you could visit a specialist.

Tics are a condition that is triggered by stress. Sleep is one of the crucial factors in the process of stress management. Your child's body does the most repair while they are asleep. It is essential for children who are struggling with broken body systems.

How much sleep is required to keep a child from being stressed? The amount of sleep required changes as your child grows. For example, a five-year-old needs sleep for about 11 hours to cope with stress for their age, while a nine-year-old needs at least ten hours of sleep to function without stress.

- Babies between four months to 12 months need at least 12 to 16 hours of sleep and naps.
- Toddlers between the ages of one to two require at least 11 to 14 hours of sleep and naps.
- Children between the ages of three to five years need ten to 13 hours of naps and sleep.
- Children between the ages of six to 12 need to sleep between nine to 12 hours.

- Teenagers require at least eight to ten hours of sleep to be free from stress and function effectively.

HOW TO HELP YOUR TEENAGE CHILD SLEEP EFFECTIVELY

Teenagers must sleep for at least eight to ten hours to have a productive and stress-free day. Here are a few tips to help your teenage child experience less stress, get enough sleep and avoid Tics:

Reduce screen time: Teenagers are likely to want to stay on their social media and have a chat with their friends instead of resting. Encouraging them to have at least an hour of free time before going to sleep will help them greatly.

Exercise: Exercise helps teenagers sleep better and improves their general health. Therefore, teenagers should always look to exercise for at least an hour every day: running, cycling, fast walking or any other aerobic activity.

Caffeine: Caffeine is a substance that is present in several beverages, such as coffee and cola. Research has shown that caffeine can prevent us from sleeping and reduce the extent of deep sleep we are likely to have. Hence, caffeine should be removed from your teenager's diet if you are looking to improve their level of sleep.

Eat moderately before bed: To get quality sleep, don't binge, as overeating will make you uncomfortable and prevent you from sleeping. You could also create a routine for sleeping and eating to help your teenage child sleep better.

Interact and talk them through their problems: You must talk to your teenage child and help him or her talk through their problems. You could also encourage the teenager to write them down if they find it difficult to communicate out loud with you. If they are given the space to voice their concerns, they are less likely to lie awake during the night worrying about them.

Chapter 13

Resting the Nervous System

The importance of resetting the nervous system cannot be overemphasized when it comes to the management of Tics. Many have argued that a Tic is a nervous condition that requires a nervous solution, while many believe that it is a muscular condition that has nothing to do with the brain. However, the causes of Tics are much more than each of those causes. Nevertheless, resetting the nervous system can be extremely helpful in the management of Tics.

The Relationship Between the Autonomic Nervous System and Tics

The nervous system has not been fully understood. Brain scans show that impaired movement activity must be examined. There is evidence showing that our sympathetic (fight or flight) and parasympathetic (rest and digest) systems may control nervous Tic activities. Fight or flight tone is mostly enhanced in patients with Tourette's syndrome compared to people without the syndrome, which often leads to changing responses. Put simply, the presence of increased fight or flight responses can be seen in most children with Tic disorders.

Nevertheless, some research has been carried out by several scientists that have helped draw a clear distinction between the fight or flight response and our ability to rest and digest.

The Relationship Between Tics, Tourette's Syndrome, and the Brain (Nervous System)

No one has a clear, distinct idea about what goes on in the human brain; however, there are several ways through which the direct relationship between the brain and Tourette's syndrome has been studied. Researchers have identified that elements known as basal ganglia are essential to the presence of Tourette's syndrome. The basal ganglia are known as a group of regions located within the core cerebral hemisphere of the brain. Many researchers and health scientists consider the basal ganglia to play a crucial role in the cognitive, emotional, and movement-related functions of a person.

This school of thought believes that inhibitory signals are received from the basal ganglia nuclei and sent to the cerebral cortex. These inhibitory signals are responsible for controlling unwanted actions such as involuntary kicking of the legs and turning of the head for no specific reason. The process of inhibition is a complex one. The same inhibitory signals that prevent unwanted movements are also responsible for the ability to restrain yourself from eating your favorite snack or holding yourself back from yelling at your boss when he or she gets on your nerves.

Just as the name implies, the inhibitory signals are responsible for the process of making sure that we don't do any of the things that we don't intend to do until we feel like doing them. It can be likened to a stopper preventing us from spilling over every time we want to.

Patients affected by Tourette's syndrome are basically dealing with a faulty inhibitory mechanism or system. The neurons that are tasked with the process of inhibiting unwanted signals from the basal ganglia fail to do what they are supposed to do. This failure leads to the execution of a habitual action such as a Tic. The failed inhibition is often accompanied by enhanced activity in motor pathways as they create a lot of movement. The patient often experiences a high level of absurd movement that creates a habitual pattern of behavior. These movements and sensory outputs are often accompanied by a very low inhibitory activity that ought to keep the pattern from playing out but has failed.

CAN YOU RESET YOUR NERVOUS SYSTEM TO DEAL WITH TICS?

There are various ways through which the nervous system can be reset to help bring stability to the rest of the body. Here are some of the ways through which the nervous system can be reset:

Resetting Through Your Breath

Breathing is literally life and is much more powerful than most people think it is. Have you ever noticed an animal that has been hunted or running for a long period of time? The animal tends to quiver and shake itself off after a while. The shaking off is often a natural response that is expected from them and acts to relieve them from drama, stress, and anxiety.

Just like the animal having escaped from its prey, we are pressed on all sides by road rage, insecurity, deadlines, taxes, or schedules which are often labeled by the nervous system as a threat to life, triggering some involuntary movement. The cumulative effect of this stressor is detrimental to one's health over time. The body remains in movement (fight or flight) throughout the stress period. As a result, the adrenaline gland is triggered, and the cortisol levels and hormonal balances are affected.

Simple steps such as breathing slowly and deeply with a consistent inhalation and exhalation ratio can help send the necessary signals to the parasympathetic parts of the nervous system to calm it down. Deep breaths serve as a tremendous help in calming down and decreasing levels of anxiety, fear, and rapid heartbeats, among other health situations. These responses have a way of influencing our physical, emotional, and mental health.

Yoga is one of the most underrated ways of resetting the nervous system. The yogic science of breathing is referred to as pranayama in the old language of Sanskrit. Pranayama is a special type of breathing that entails the use of observation, expansion, control, and the adjustment of your breath to enhance the longevity, vitality, and life force of the body. It also helps boost memory, as well as enhance the circulation and oxygenation of the blood. A subsequent study showed that the physical and cognitive benefits that yoga provides may be due to the deep pranayama breathing which can activate the parasympathetic nervous system.

You can guide your child through all or some of these processes to help them reset their nerves.

Before you start, ensure you sit in a comfortable position or in a chair to ensure that you are able to go the distance and achieve the result you are looking for.

Once you start: It is important that you breathe in with your abdomen, fill the air and expand while you breathe out, and try to empty your abdomen on the out breath. If your system is stressed, you might have to inhale and see your abdomen move inwards and exhale while your abdomen moves outwards. The reverse action of the system should be to expand the abdomen, exhale and contract the abdomen; it is vital that all of this should be done on an empty stomach.

Studying the breath and Sama Vritti: There are practices that are meditational, such as vipassana, that have a history of helping people get the best out of their systems. Focusing your attention on your breath fixates the mind on one point and helps you get the best out of it by easing the distractions of a wandering mind that can boost the heart rate of an individual or cause anxiety.

To do this, you could simply begin by studying your breath as you inhale in and out. Maintain the rhythm while you try to study the movement and feel the part of the nose where the air is passing through and over. Then after five breaths, you simply begin to inhale for a count of four and exhale for four. This technique helps to relieve stress, anxiety, or any form of agitation. Once an equal ratio has been established, you could try increasing the ratio to six or eight.

The Complete Breath (Dirgha Pranayama): This type of breath is designed to fill all three aspects of the lungs and help remove any toxicity from the blood and enhance deep oxygenation. It helps eliminate shallow chest breathing and cultivates a deeper and longer breathing pattern, which helps in digestion and in optimizing circulation.

This pranayama is also known as a three-part breath that has an inhalation that should be practiced in a uniform and continuous complete breath. To carry out this practice, it is important that the fingers point towards the abdomen. The nostrils then can inhale slowly and expand the abdomen, inflating it. As you inhale, slide your palms up your rib cage and bring them to rest on your collarbone. Slowly draw in the lower part of the abdomen till the chest is full.

Hold your breath for a few seconds and exhale through the nostrils again. This time, place the palms on the chest, press your hands on the torso and slide them down as you breathe out at each section slowly. As a result, the abdomen is expected to be drawn in and lifted upwards while you exhale. You can repeat the process up to nine times if you like.

If you are feeling dizzy at any point, you could lie down while carrying out this breathing exercise. You could also stop the entire process if the dizziness persists. Only do as much as you or your child are comfortable with.

Alternate nostril breathing: This process is often referred to as Nadi Shodhana but is most known as alternate nostril breathing. This technique is great for cleansing and balancing - bringing homeostasis to the nervous system. It is best to practice this type of breathing in the morning to be able to take charge of the day. This approach is also used in yoga and some other types of meditation processes.

To carry this out, place your left hand on your left knee and find a comfortable posture. Take your right hand and bend the index finger and middle finger across your palm. After assuming this hand position, try exhaling out your nostrils. After the exhale has been completed, close the right nostril with your thumb while you inhale through your left nostril.

Change over to closing your left nostril and exhaling through the right nostril. Then breathe in through the right nostril. This process should be repeated about seven times.

Deep Sigh

Taking deep sighs is one of the ways the nervous system can be reset. To achieve a deep sigh, you must deeply breathe in and breathe out for longer. Research has shown that deep sighs move the autonomic nervous system from an over-activated state (which cannot be curbed by inhibitors) to a balanced and stable parasympathetic state.

Deep sighs not only reset the nervous system but also help give you a clear and calm head, helping you to respond effectively to whatever happens next.

Touch

The nervous system works hand in hand with the senses of trust and touch. Touch is another method you can use to reset your nervous system. Safe touch helps to activate oxytocin which generates a cooling effect on the human brain, creating a calm feeling, and serving as an antidote to cortisol, the stress hormone. Oxytocin is also one of the series of neurochemicals that are part of the brain and play a crucial role in social engagement.

Placing Hands on the Heart

Studies have also shown that placing your hands on your heart helps soothe the mind and helps reset the nervous system. It also helps develop a sense of security which helps release oxytocin to help fight stress.

Movement

Movement often helps people to improve their mood by activating the autonomic nervous system. Research has shown that altering the posture of your body can also alter your mood.

The steps above are not only capable of boosting the inhibitors but are also capable of resetting the nervous system. Since Tics are associated with stress, fear, and anxiety, calming your nerves is vital when dealing with Tics and Tourette's syndrome.

COMPLEMENTARY APPROACHES

Behavioral Therapies

Behavioral therapy is often a common treatment of Tics. It is like psychological therapy in that a specialist psychologist is required. Habit reversal therapy is one of the major therapies used in the treatment of Tics. Habit reversal therapy aims to:

- Educate you about your condition.
- Help you identify when your Tic occurs, the urges that accompany it, and the triggers.
- Give you information about the appropriate response when the urge that accompanies the Tic begins. For instance, if your Tic makes you shrug your shoulder, you might have to stretch your hands to deal with the experience till the Tic passes.

In severe cases, Comprehensive Behavioral Intervention for Tics (CBIT) may be utilized. This is when a series of behavioral techniques are employed to reduce the occurrence of Tics. Another technique referred to as Exposure and Response Prevention (ERP) is also used to deal with Tics. This technique focuses on helping you reduce the feeling and the embarrassment that comes with Tics till the experience passes.

Despite the effectiveness of these techniques, they require several sessions with a therapist and must be used continuously even after the treatment is completed. Although they can be effective in managing symptoms you may want to use them in conjunction with functional lab testing to look deeper at what is going on inside the body.

Acupuncture

Acupuncture can be a great complementary approach for Tic disorders. Some of the benefits are that acupuncture:

- is very specific for the treatment of Tic disorders
- diminishes stress
- can reduce anxiety around Tics or their anticipation

The use of acupuncture in the treatment of Tic disorders was first introduced by Dr. J.R. Worsley, an Australian, who found acupuncture to be effective for some individuals with Tourette's syndrome. The results gained from acupuncture were so dramatic that they resulted in more than an 80 percent improvement. Since then, there have been other reports on success stories with this therapy among both children and adults (Alonso-Alonso et al., 2009). Even though acupuncture is relatively new as a complementary approach to Tic disorders, the therapy has been around for thousands of years. Acupuncture often incorporates Chinese medicine into the practice to help balance the body. The acupuncture point associated with Tourette's syndrome is "Guan Yuan" ("Gates of Consciousness"). This name was chosen because it is located near where Tics commonly occur. According to acupuncture theory, people who have Tourette's syndrome are thought to have an imbalance in their energy or qi. This "qi" is very important because it is said to regulate all the systems in the body,

Chiropractic Care

Chiropractic care has been shown to reduce both the severity and frequency of symptoms associated with Tic disorders. This makes sense because the spine and nervous system are interrelated. The central nervous system (CNS) controls and coordinates all functions of the entire body, including Tics; when there is a decreased function in the CNS, Tic symptoms can be exacerbated. Chiropractors believe that Tic symptoms can worsen if there is a misalignment in the spine, so chiropractic care can help relieve some Tic symptoms by realigning the spine and allowing the CNS to operate more smoothly.

The Vagus nerve may also play a role when it comes to misalignment. The Vagus nerve is the longest cranial nerve, stretching all the way from the brain to the abdomen. It helps control functions of the face and neck muscles, stomach, heart, lungs, kidney function, liver function, blood pressure regulation, and maybe even Tics themselves.

Is a chiropractor the magic bullet? Although some people have had success with chiropractic care for Tics, many have found it will not ultimately make them go away but it can help reduce symptoms. There are many layers of Tic disorders, and poor alignment may be one of the contributing factors but is most likely not the main problem. Chiropractic care can be a great complementary approach when managing Tic disorders.

Supplements

I want to touch on using supplements as an approach to Tic disorders. Somehow when we do a Google search on Tic disorders, supplements tend to be the first thing to pop up. Those recommendations include things like magnesium and vitamin B6. In my research and experience, I have not found anybody to clearly state that Tic disorders are caused by a nutritional deficiency. It may be one of the contributing factors, but supplements are not a magic bullet for making them go away.

Supplements are meant to supplement, not replace, a healthy diet and lifestyle. Make sure you are doing everything you can to develop a healthy lifestyle before you add in supplements. It is important to note too that not all supplements are equally effective and that many of them contain fillers and ingredients that are not a great choice for your child with a Tic disorder. While magnesium and B6 will probably not hurt them, they are not the most common nutrient deficiency I see in my clients. I can tell you from experience that most of the clients who come to me and have previously tried magnesium and B6 feel like they didn't do much good. Therefore, it is extremely important to test not guess. When we test, we can create an individualized plan based on the exact needs of your child. When you have an individualized plan, you no longer need to play guessing games by trying to use supplements, certain diets or prescriptions. The plan tells you what supplements your child needs in the right dose at the right time.

Try to Take Your Mind off the Tic When Experiencing a Flare

Many times, children will experience an increase in Tics. This can be due to illness, stress, and even exhaustion. Many parents want to know how to deal with a flare when it does occur.

The trick is simply not to draw too much attention and make the condition worse. If the condition is known to the child, there are chances they will develop unnecessary anxiety and stress, thereby worsening the situation. It is also important that you draw a line between this and outrightly ignoring the child when needed. You must keep a watch over the child and notice serious changes whenever they arise.

Ultimately, the aim is to make certain that the child is calm and assure them that all will be well. Your job is to calm the child down, boost their self-esteem, and save them from embarrassment through your interaction. You could also engage the child in necessary activities to help them take their mind off the situation, such as deep breaths.

How to Deal with a Tic Flair

Here are a few things to avoid to help you better deal with the severity of the symptoms of Tics:

Fitness and Exercise: Exercise helps us to produce neurotransmitters and also helps to get our bowels moving. It helps young children to use energy and sleep peacefully, so their nervous systems can reset at the same time. Furthermore, the participation of young children in group activities such as volleyball or soccer (but really any sport will do), can help boost their self-esteem. Exercise is a stress reliever, and many families see a reduction in Tics when their child gets regular exercise.

Reduce Sugar Intake: This is a crucial part of effective dieting as it includes reducing natural sugars themselves. You could try out the ketogenic approach to

mitigate the symptoms of Tics. A decrease in sugar consumption has been known to help deal with neurological issues, like Tourette's. This implies that you must completely cut out things like juices and sodas from the diet and also drastically reduce the consumption of fruits, which contain a large number of natural sugars.

Abstain from gluten: Going gluten-free has proven to help reduce the symptoms of Tics. Increase your vegetable intake and reduce gluten. Simple.

Reduce your screen time: A relationship has been found between the amount of screen time experienced and the frequency at which people have their Tics, so it is essential that you reduce the amount of time you allow your child to spend on the screens.

Relax: Yoga, meditation, and deep breathing can also help when your child experiences a flair. Refer to earlier in the book for some detailed relaxation methods.

Sleep: Sleep and rest are key for the body to regenerate. Make sure that your child is getting at least eight to ten hours of sleep every night. If your teenager sleeps all day, it's OK, they are growing and they need it. Trust me, I'm a mom with two teenagers.

PART 3

Relieving the Burden

Chapter 14

Connecting the Dots

Now that you have looked at the formula, it's time to really connect the dots.

Let's start at the beginning of my story with my son, Whit, so that you can clearly see the story as it unfolds.

Whit's food sensitivity test showed several sensitivities to gluten, dairy, peanuts, eggs, and soy. We had previously removed some of the offenders like gluten and dairy, but having this extra data helped refine his diet further. The blood work showed that Whit did have a previous Epstein Barr infection, and the functional lab testing pulled up some even more surprising results. His heavy metal and environmental results showed super high levels of uranium which I attribute to the fact that an atomic bomb had been blown up in New Mexico. His stool pathogen test showed elevated levels of candida, leaky gut, and an imbalanced microbiome. Finally, gene testing showed a predisposition to chronic inflammation, poor detoxification, glutamate sensitivity, nutrient deficiency, and gluten intolerance.

The first step was to put all these pieces together. We knew that he had all these layers of issues in the body, and we needed to approach them one by one to avoid getting overwhelmed.

First, we tackled diet. It was essential for us to stick to a whole-food, paleo-style diet. And since the only Nutritionist in town was booked solid for six months, I was left to my own devices. I collected cookbooks, scoured Pinterest, and created many of my own recipes (some of which I will share with you later in this book). I also made sure that Whit was drinking clean, filtered water. Finally, we cut out the junk and sugar.

Next, we used his genes as a roadmap to ensure that he was getting enough nutrients based on his genetics, and we were able to create a supplement plan based on his needs. We knew that he needed extra vitamin D, folate, B12, and an anti-inflammatory protocol based on his genes. He was already on an anti-inflammatory diet, so we added some anti-inflammatory supplements that included omega-3 fatty acids, CBD oil, and Palmitoylethanolamide (PEA). PEA is stellar for reducing neural inflammation, pain, and swelling. Keep in mind that we introduced everything in a specific order and very slowly. We also started doing glutathione IVs to help with detoxification as his detox pathways do not work well genetically and we knew he had an abundance of uranium in his system. Children with Tics are sensitive, and we did not want to overload his system.

We were on our way, and we needed to give Whit a little time to settle before we worked on the gut. Our alternative allergist was great and helped us balance the candida overgrowth with a prescription for nystatin. If you cannot find a doctor to prescribe nystatin, other natural approaches include certain supplements like Saccharomyces Boulardii, Biocidin, Berberine, and garlic. We did not initially add in a probiotic because many children with Tics experience an increase when a probiotic is introduced. Stool pathogen testing can guide you when selecting targeted probiotics to address the exact issues in the gut.

Getting rid of all processed foods was vital for improving Whit's sleep. Glutamates are very excitatory to the brain; they can cause an increase in Tics and an inability to initiate sleep. At least 90% of the packaged, processed foods in your grocery store are full of glutamates. They are put there as a chemical to keep us coming back for more. Monosodium glutamate is a form of glutamate that is the most known. The USDA says that companies can put MSG in any food if it is less than 99% pure. When it is less than 99% pure, they can call it whatever they want. I have provided you with a copy of my glutamate list at the end of this book.

Once you have been infected with the Epstein-Barr (EBV) virus, it lays dormant in your DNA, waiting to be triggered by environmental factors like viruses, toxins, chemicals in food, or artificial sweeteners. When EBV is triggered (or reactivated), it can cause fatigue and migraines both before and during the active virus stage of infection. So we know that we have to keep Whit healthy and his inflammation down so that he does not experience a flair of EBV. All the approaches we were using, and still use today, give his body the best environment for keeping EBV at bay.

Exercise was a significant factor for Whit, and we had to ensure he got plenty of it. Exercise can be critical for children with Tic disorders. It has tons of positive impacts on physical and mental health as well as Tic symptoms. For example, intense physical activity helps release endorphins in the body, which help provide natural stress relief. It also allowed Whit to sleep better at night.

We removed all the toxins from our home. We got rid of plastics, anything scented, and harsh cleaners like bleach. We also swapped our creams, lotions, toothpaste, shampoo, conditioner, and soaps with nontoxic, clean versions. Finally, we switched to green cleaners like hot water, vinegar, and lemons.

We also incorporated meditation, deep breathing, chiropractic care, and acupuncture to help rebalance Whit's nervous system. These complementary approaches enabled him to relax and get his body out of flight or fight mode.

The number one question I get asked is, "How soon after you made all these changes did you see Tics improve?" I will tell you that the results are very different for everybody I work with, but for us, we had already started making a lot of these changes along the way. The genetic testing was one of the last functional lab tests we did, and once we incorporated genetics and used those results to create a roadmap, we saw tremendous results in about 30 days. We were doing occupational therapy for his sensory disorders during the time that we incorporated with the genetic approach. After six occupational therapy sessions, he got kicked out, and we were told he no longer qualified because the changes we made for him caused drastic improvements in his sensory issues. Keep in mind that this is not usually typical. We had done a lot of the other work beforehand.

It has been ten years since Whit was diagnosed, and we still use 99% of these approaches in our home. His genetic test frequently sits on my desk, and I refer to it regularly. It indeed has been a roadmap for us and a fantastic way for us to connect the dots with all the functional lab testing and his symptoms. This process has taught Whit to listen to his body, and he can tell you that it impacts his brain and gut when he cheats on his diet. He is Tic-free 99.9% of the time unless we have some underlying infection that causes inflammation. You have heard me mention that Tics are the boil-over symptom, they are what we see on the outside after imbalance has already taken place on the inside. We know if we see any form of Tic that we need to look deeper, his check engine light is on, and we need to figure out what is going on.

Chapter 15

Tic Relief Is Possible

Before we reach the end of this book, I want to share with you some real-life examples of what is possible for you when you approach your child's Tic disorder using my Comprehensive Neuro-Immune Analysis formula.

Now I'm All Better.

When I was little, I wanted to be a doctor. I thought helping people get better would be the noblest and most rewarding profession. In time, I realized that doctor's hours were just not going to work for me. What I wanted to be even more than a doctor, was a mom (and yes, many women do both – they are superheroes!). So, my career took a different, yet wonderful turn. I became a teacher, quite by accident, but it suited me perfectly. I found that I am an educator at heart and taught Spanish and French for 13 years at the secondary level. I loved every minute of working with students and families, teaching them, and learning from them.

Life did what it does, bringing new opportunities and choices to be made. It's funny how things come full circle. Now, here I am, a few babies and a global pandemic later, working for Dr. Gibson, helping people get better! I guess the little girl version of me got her wish after all. I now get to combine my years of experience in education and advocacy as well as my knowledge of health and wellness to teach others AND help them get better.

I specialize in family health, and I am the go-to-gal for your dietary and lifestyle changes as you work through your protocol with Dr. Gibson. I help with recipe revamps, brand recommendations, pantry cleanouts, grocery lists, label reading, and more. I also write blogs for Dr. Gibson based on topics that are generated within our Facebook group (Tic Disorder Secrets: A Natural Approach) or through client surveys.

Another part of my job that I am very committed to is taking initial consult calls. I love getting to know people, I am a great listener, and I take notes at the speed of light (#teacherskills). I am so grateful for technology and our ability to connect with people in different states, countries, time zones, and on different continents. I meet with families whose children are going through what my daughter went through. I hear their struggles, their sadness, and their despair. I can empathize with what they are experiencing because I have been in their shoes. As moms and dads ask me through tears, "Does this really get better?" I can confidently say, "Yes, it absolutely does," because I have lived through it. It gets better. There is hope.

Let me tell you our story.

My daughter was diagnosed with OCD, anxiety, sensory processing disorder, mood swings, and ADHD between the ages of two and six. She received the diagnosis of Tourette's syndrome at the age of seven. I was prepared for it; I already knew what the doctor would say from my Google searches. Of course, I came armed with my questions about medications and natural approaches, dietary adjustments and more. In the end, the doctor could only prescribe medication and did not give much merit to parent reports about holistic ways to manage symptoms.

At first, we tried to change her diet by eliminating food dyes, and it did help a little, but not enough. We tried many medications and saw countless doctors including neurologists, ENTs, ophthalmologists, ophthalmology specialists, occupational therapists, psychologists, and dermatologists, and attended a CBIT clinic four or five times a week for months on end. We exercised, tried yoga, and belly breathing, ignored Tics, talked about Tics and tried vitamins and supplements. Nothing was working and she was only getting worse.

People always ask if I can share my daughter's symptoms. It's hard to write about what she went through even now that she is Tic-free, and these symptoms are gone. She went through hell. Looking back, I don't even know how she still managed to enjoy life. It was heartbreaking.

Her symptoms included: severe vocal and motor Tics, stomach pain, nausea, nightmares, separation anxiety (particularly at bedtime or when going to school), outbursts, impulsive behavior, frustration and fits, anger, intrusive thoughts, compulsions, fear of death, social skill deficits, falling behind in school, lack of concentration, inability to complete multi-step tasks without frequent redirection and/or direct supervision, getting "stuck" in a sequence, needing everything to be "just so", rituals (before bed, before leaving a room, etc.), repetition of words and phrases, unexplained body pains (bones, skin, eyelashes), constipation, diarrhea, bloating, gas, cramps, heavy menstrual cycles, extreme fatigue, dizziness, weakness, brain fog, depression, suicidal ideations, rashes, itching, flushing, sweating, feeling hot and cold chills, inability to tolerate loud noises, bright lights, jeans, or certain textures, and I'm sure as soon as I publish this I will think of a list of things I forgot to add.

Can I take a moment to remind you that my daughter was 7–13 years old and experiencing all of these symptoms? She would say, "Mama, I feel like my body is so old."

The breaking point was the night that she came into my room and laid down on my bed and said words that shook me to my core. "I don't want to live like this anymore." Sheer terror raced through me. As a teacher, I have lost students to suicide. I'm trained to know what to look and listen for. I told my daughter that we would find a solution and she would get better. I made her sleep in my room that night for fear that she might hurt herself. And I lay awake, scouring the internet, I resolved to find someone who could help us. My daughter is under the care of a psychologist who we contacted immediately.

If you are in crisis or think you may have an emergency, call your doctor or 911 immediately. If you're having suicidal thoughts, call 1-800-273-TALK (8255) to talk to a skilled, trained counselor at a crisis center in your area at any time (National Suicide Prevention Lifeline). If you are located outside the United States, call your local emergency line immediately.

I was referred to Dr. Gibson by another mom in a Facebook group. After our initial consult call, I was optimistically skeptical – if that's a thing. This lady was telling me that my child could get better. I wanted to believe her, I NEEDED to believe her because I was desperate, and we had tried everything. I was out of options, out of ideas, and I needed a new approach. If anyone was going to be able to help my daughter, it was Dr. Gibson. So, we took a leap of faith and committed wholeheartedly to the process.

Dr. Gibson's approach was the opposite of everything I had ever heard of before. She was looking for the root cause and scientific proof about what was going on under the surface for my daughter. She was the first person to look at my daughter as a whole person rather than a list of individual symptoms.

Dr. Gibson will probably laugh at what I'm about to say. Do you know the character Grandmother Willow in the Disney movie Pocahontas? Remember how she was all, "Listen to the earth" and "Sometimes the right way is not the easiest one"? Well, folks, that's Dr. Gibson. She listens to the body and does not guarantee that the path is an easy one. BUT SHE GETS YOU ON THE RIGHT PATH FOR YOU.

People always ask me how long it took to start seeing changes in my daughter. The answer is after a while and all at once. Within two weeks certain symptoms started to subside and disappear. I didn't even realize that certain things were getting better until I spoke to Dr. Gibson about eight weeks into our protocol and I was worrying because my daughter was still ticking. Dr. Gibson assured me that things would improve and reminded me that her body had a lot of healing to do, from the inside out.

And then we hit 90 days in. AND. THE. TICS. WERE. GONE. I came downstairs and surprisingly found my child "chilling" on the sofa watching TV before school. She never had extra time. This is a kid who was usually still pulling her socks and shoes on while hopping on one foot at a time on the way to the car. This is not an "extra time before school" child that I have. I tried to play it cool. "Hey, honey, you're done early..." awkward pause as her eyes finally fluttered away from the TV. "Oh, yeah I had SO much extra time because I wasn't ticking." JUST. LIKE. THAT. I think I managed to say, "Oh that's awesome!" but my mind was like "Don't jinx it, don't talk about it." Can I just say the lack of noise from my child was eerie? It was utterly unnerving taking her to school with no sounds coming from the back seat. I didn't even tell Dr. Gibson right away. It was like in grade school when you don't say "snow" because superstitiously it might scare the snow away. I was afraid that this was a fluke. Surely, when I picked her up from school that day the Tics would be back ...

Guess what?

It's been four months. The Tics are still gone. And every other symptom is gone, too. Readers, my child – for the first time in her life – wore jeans two weeks ago. This is something I didn't even list on my wish list of symptoms to magically get rid of.

After seeing the drastic changes in my daughter, a new passion is ignited in me. I feel absolutely compelled to share my experience with other families who feel that there is no hope, no answer, or no way out of the storm of symptoms they are plagued with.

Not everyone I talk to believes me. Some people have questioned my motives for promoting Dr. Gibson so wholeheartedly. Yes, I work for her now, but that is not the reason I want to bring every child with Tics or a laundry list of symptoms into her program.

It's because I witnessed a miracle. And I must tell everyone. I can't keep this to myself.

My daughter, who has attended a special private school for children with learning disabilities since she was diagnosed with TS, had lofty hopes of attending a local high school with a theater program.

Guess what?

She got in! And she was awarded a Presidential Scholarship for Voice!

She was invited to try out for our local rock-climbing team.

Guess what?

She made it! She even set a record for climbing a wall six times in five minutes. Being timed used to be such a source of anxiety and always used to cause more Tics. Not now!

With Dr. Gibson's help, I have given my daughter the tools she needs to make educated and responsible choices for her health as she grows into an adult. Yes, it is a daily choice for her to stay on track with her protocol. Occasionally, my daughter chooses to veer off the path. She is learning how foods and stress affect her body, how much of something is too much and what she can tolerate.

There are points in your life where, in hindsight, you realize you were at a fork in your path. The direction you chose to go at that time altered everything that came after.

I chose Dr. Gibson; against the advice of some people that I hold near and dear to my heart. Not everyone had the faith that I had. Not everyone understood why I was trusting a lady who lived across the country from me and who I'd never met in person. People I love fought with me and tried to change my mind! I stuck to my guns.

Times have changed. Technology allows us access to experts who don't live nearby. I vetted Dr. Gibson with another mom who had an amazing story and that was that. I chose the path of an unfamiliar approach, and it was a bit intimidating, but I knew it was the right choice for us.

I am so glad I took the risk.

I have my girl back. She is happy, a total chatterbox, more tolerant, more balanced, Tic free, has manageable menstrual cycles, has regular BMs, and she is just enjoying being a kid. She loves singing, theater, and doing makeup. She is an even bigger Dr. Gibson promoter than I am! She has actually gotten on a few initial consult calls to tell people firsthand that THIS PROCESS WORKS. Her life has changed.

Recently, I asked her to describe to me a little bit about her process with Dr. Gibson and I asked if there was anything she wanted other kids who might be considering working with Dr. Gibson to know.

I'll end with my daughter's testimony."

"Dr. Gibson is nice. She helps you know what you can eat. The biggest help for me was the food part of it. I didn't know certain things were making me worse. Now I can move my body because I WANT to not because I HAVE to. I used to Tic all the time."

"And how about now?"

"Now I'm all better."

-Danielle M. Goetzinger

My mom gut knew something was off

As a mother and a pharmacist, I can't sing Piper's praises enough. She is incredible to work with and will treat your kids as her own.

My son experienced a few Tic "episodes" following illnesses and I was told they were normal and just a coincidence of the timing. My mom gut knew something was off. My own research told me we were dealing with other issues. I started supplements from my own research and saw some improvement, but I wanted concrete answers. Piper validated my thoughts both as a mom and as a holistic practitioner. Through genetic testing, stool analysis, food sensitivities, and a very detailed history we found the root causes.

After some adjustments and streamlining supplements specific to my son's results – we have a new gut and a much healthier immune system and no longer deal with Tics after infections.

A year down the line I found myself having issues with Raynaud's phenomenon and a positive ANA which is an autoimmune marker.

I immediately reached out to Piper and after a careful history and some lab work, she suggested some supplements for me. After a few weeks, I had incredible results. I have not had a Raynaud's "attack" (even in a Northeast winter full of snow) and my ANA is no longer positive.

Piper creates a personalized plan based on your history and it's not a one-size-fits-all. Her knowledge is remarkable, and her passion is contagious to help families.

My only regret was not partnering with her sooner.

As a board-certified pharmacotherapy specialist, I am incredibly impressed with Piper's execution in navigating various health conditions."

Ashley Kapanek Pharm.D., BCPS

Chapter 16

Recipes

Food is one of the most important factors that determines good health. The impact of good and healthy food cannot be overemphasized on the well-being of every individual, particularly young children. Tourette's patients, or children suffering from Tics, cannot overlook such an important factor in dealing with their condition. As a mother just starting out and making diet changes I was overwhelmed and stressed. I want you to have some tools you can incorporate into your journey right away.

Breakfast

BAILEY'S HOMEMADE GLUTEN FREE "FLOUR" TORTILLAS

These are great for breakfast tacos!

Diet Type: Gluten-free, Dairy free, Egg-free

Ingredients:

1½ cups Bob's Red Mill 1 tol Gluten Free Baking Mix
½ teaspoon baking powder
½ teaspoon salt
2 tablespoons lard or solidified bacon grease
(that's what I usually use)
¾ cup ice water

Method:

1. Whisk together flour, salt, and baking soda.
2. Use your hands to work in the lard/grease. Make sure no large pieces remain.
3. Add ½ cup ice water (no ice) and stir with a spoon. Slowly add the last quarter of water. If it holds together and feels damp, stop adding water.
4. Flour your countertop. Knead dough until smooth.
5. Pull off some dough and roll it into balls. Smash flat and roll out to a thin tortilla.
6. Heat cast iron over medium heat.
7. Place the tortilla into the skillet to brown. Flip it to cook both sides.

WATERMELON SMOOTHIE

Diet Type: GF, DF, egg-free, paleo, classic, vegan

Ingredients:

1 cup coconut water or almond milk
2 tablespoons lemon juice
2 mint leaves
1 tablespoon chia seeds
1½ cups watermelon chunks, frozen
1 tablespoon coconut oil

Method:

1. Place all ingredients into a blender.
2. Blend well until smooth.
3. Divide into glasses and enjoy!

BLUEBERRY SMOOTHIE

Diet Type: GF, DF, egg-free, paleo, classic, vegan

Ingredients:

1 cup coconut water or almond milk
2 tablespoons lemon juice
2 mint leaves
1 tablespoon chia seeds
1½ cups watermelon chunks, frozen
1 tablespoon coconut oil

Method:

1. Place all ingredients into a blender.
2. Blend well until smooth.
3. Divide into glasses and enjoy!

KIWI SMOOTHIE BOWL

Diet Type: GF, DF, egg-free, paleo, classic, vegan

Ingredients:

½ cup dairy-free milk
2 kiwis, chopped
1 large frozen banana, chopped
1 cup mixed greens
1 scoop protein powder (we use grass-fed beef protein)
1 tablespoon flax seeds
¼ cup blueberries

Method:

1. Add all ingredients except flax seeds to a blender.
2. Blend until smooth.
3. Serve in a bowl topped with flax seeds and blueberries.

CHIA SEED PUDDING

Diet Type: GF, DF, egg-free, classic, paleo

Ingredients:

3 tbsps. chia seeds
¾ cup unsweetened almond milk
¼ tsp cinnamon
1 apple or pear (cored and diced)
2 tbsps. pecans
1 tbsp almond butter

Method:

1. Whisk together the chia seeds, almond milk and cinnamon in a small pot over medium-low heat.
2. Stir until heated through and the mixture has thickened up - about 5 to 7 minutes.
3. Remove from heat and add to a bowl. Top with apples, pecans, and almond butter.

SAUSAGE GRAVY

Diet type: Classic, GF, DF, egg-free, paleo

Ingredients:

1 tbsp extra virgin olive oil
1 garlic clove (minced)
1 sweet onion (medium, chopped)
1 lb. nitrate-free Sausage (you can substitute bacon)
Sea salt to taste
1 tsp. black pepper
1 cup organic coconut milk or another dairy substitute
1 tsp arrowroot powder

Method:

1. Heat olive oil in a large skillet over medium heat. Cook the garlic and onion for about 5 minutes or until translucent.
2. Add the sausage, salt, and pepper. Use a spatula to stir and break up the sausage as it cooks. Sauté until cooked through. Stir in coconut milk and arrowroot powder.
3. Cook for about 5 to 10 minutes, or until the mixture has thickened. Taste and adjust seasoning if needed.

SAUSAGE AND APPLES

Diet type: Classic, GF, DF, egg-free, paleo

Ingredients:

8 oz nitrate-free beef or pork sausage (sliced)
1 apple (cored, chopped)
1 onion, sliced
1 tsp cinnamon½ avocado (pitted, halved)

Method:

1. Place a large skillet over medium heat.
2. Add the sausage, onion, apples, and cinnamon.
3. Cook for 8 to 10 minutes, or until the sausage is cooked through and the apples are soft. Substitute apples with pear or you can also use chorizo, chicken, pork, or vegan sausage.

Lunch/Dinner

DILL CHICKEN

Diet Type: Classic, Paleo, DF, GF

Ingredients:

½ cup mayonnaise
Salt/pepper to taste
1 tbsp fresh dill1 lb. chicken thighs
(bone-in, skin removed)

Method:

1. Preheat the oven to 400ºF (204ºC) and line a baking sheet with parchment paper.
2. Add the mayonnaise and dill into a small bowl. Whisk together until evenly combined.
3. Add the chicken to the sauce and toss until well-coated.
4. Transfer the chicken onto the baking sheet and cook for 25 to 30 minutes or until cooked through.

GLAZED RIBS

Diet Type: AIP, GF, DF, egg-free, grain-free, paleo, soy-free

Ingredients:

¼ cup coconut aminos
2 tbsp fish sauce
3 tbsp maple syrup
½ yellow onion (chopped)
1 tsp ginger (peeled, chopped)
4 garlic cloves (minced)
2 green onions (chopped, divided)3 lb. pork ribs

Method:

1. In a bowl, make your marinade by whisking together the coconut aminos, fish sauce, maple syrup, onion, ginger, garlic and green onion.
2. Place your ribs in the slow cooker and brush the marinade on all sides. Cook on low for 6 to 8 hours, or high for 4 hours.
3. When ready to eat, preheat the grill over medium heat.
4. Carefully remove the ribs from the slow cooker onto a plate. Grill for 10 minutes per side, or until slightly charred. Brush with any remaining marinade while grilling.

WHOLE ROASTED CHICKEN

Diet Type: Classic, Paleo, Keto, GF, DF, egg-free,

Serves 6

Ingredients:

1 large white onion, cut into thick slices
1 5–6 lb. whole chicken
Sea salt, to taste
1 tbsp. poultry seasoning
¼ cup tallow or lard, warmed
6–8 cloves garlic, finely minced, divided
1 cup chicken broth

Method:

1. Preheat oven to 425 °F and arrange onion slices in the bottom of a large, heavy-duty 12" roaster with high sides.
2. Remove the neck and giblets from the chicken and boil them on low for giblet gravy or for your pets. Don't let them go to waste.
3. Prepare the bird. Place bird breast side up on top of onion slices in skillet. Pat chicken dry with paper towels and generously rub it with tallow. Next season the outside with poultry seasoning and minced garlic. You may even want to tuck some of the tallow and seasoning under the skin. Add the broth and garlic to the pan.
4. Place skillet in preheated oven and roast for 1 hour and 30 minutes or until a meat thermometer inserted into the thickest part of the thigh reads 165° F. Check every 30 minutes while cooking to make sure the skin isn't becoming too brown. If it is becoming too brown turn the oven down.
5. Remove the skillet from the oven and let rest for 15-20 minutes.
6. While the chicken rests, discard the onion slices in the skillet and heat the remaining liquid over medium-high heat. Scrape the bottom of the roaster with a spatula or wooden spoon to remove the browned bits. Continue cooking until the liquid is reduced by one-half. Once reduced, taste and season with salt, if desired. You can use this for gravy on a side of potatoes.

TURKEY AND RICE ZUCCHINI BOATS

Diet Type: GF, DF, Classic, egg-free

Ingredients:

¼ cup steamed white non-enriched white rice
2 zucchinis
1½ tbsps. extra virgin olive oil
1 yellow onion (diced)
1 pound ground turkey
½ red bell pepper (diced)
¼cup black pepper
¼tsp. sea salt
1½ tsp. tamari
1 tsp garlic

Method:

1. Preheat oven to 350°F (177°C).
2. Trim the ends off the zucchini. Cut zucchini in half lengthwise and scoop out the pulp using a teaspoon. Finely chop the pulp.
3. In a large skillet, heat olive oil over medium heat. Add onion, garlic, ground turkey, zucchini pulp, red bell pepper, black pepper, and sea salt. Stir until turkey is cooked through (8 to 10 minutes).
4. When turkey is cooked, drain the skillet of excess juice and stir in tamari and cooked rice. Remove from heat.
5. Spoon turkey rice filling into the zucchini shells. Bake in the oven for 20 minutes or until the zucchini is tender.

TACOS

Diet type: Classic, GF, DF, egg-free

Ingredients:

8 ORGANIC** corn tortillas
1 tbsp avocado oil
1 lb. grass-fed ground beef
½ tsp onion powder
½ tsp garlic powder
½ tsp paprika
½ tsp sea salt
½ tsp cumin
½ head green lettuce (small, finely chopped)
2 tomatoes (medium, diced)

Method:

1. Prepare tortillas according to instructions on the package.
2. Heat a large skillet over medium heat. Add the avocado oil and the beef, stirring to break it up as it cooks.
3. Add the onion powder, paprika, garlic powder, salt, and cumin to the pan. Once the beef is cooked through, remove it from the heat.
4. Add the ground beef, lettuce, and tom.

**Unless it is ORGANIC corn is genetically modified and full of toxins.

Treats

ALMOND BANANA BOAT

Diet Type: GF, DF, paleo, vegan, egg-free, classic

Ingredients:

1tbsp. almond butter or any nut butter
½ tbsp water (warm)
1 banana (peeled)
1 tbsp. unsweetened shredded coconut

Method:

1. In a small bowl, whisk the almond butter and water together until all lumps disappear and a thin consistency is reached.
2. Slice the banana lengthwise or into coins.
3. Drizzle with almond butter and sprinkle the shredded coconut overtop.

CLEAN TRAIL MIX

Diet type: vegan, paleo, classic, DF, GF, egg-free

Ingredients:

½ cup pumpkin seeds
½ cup pistachios
½ cup sunflower seeds
½ cup cashews
½ cups almonds
½ cup pecans
½ cup raisins or craisins

Method:

1. Mix in an airtight container
2. Remove the dried fruit for keto

GRILLED FRUIT

Diet Type: Classic, GF, GF, egg-free, paleo, primal

Ingredients:

2 cups pineapple (diced and cored)
1 cup strawberries (halved and stems removed)
1 peach (sliced and pit removed)
6 apricots
12 barbecue skewers
1 cup blueberries¼ lime (juiced)

Method:

1. Preheat grill to high heat.
2. Slide the pineapple, strawberries, apricots, and nectarine onto skewers. (Note: If using wooden skewers, they should be soaked in water beforehand.)
3. Grill fruit skewers for 1 to 2 minutes per side, or until grill marks appear.
4. Slide the grilled fruit off the skewers and into a bowl. Add the blueberries, top with lime juice and enjoy!
5. Recipes That Can Be Made from Flaxseed

FLAXSEED SMOOTHIE

A flaxseed smoothie is a common smoothie rich in omega 3, a drink low in calories, and a great source of fiber. The drink can be prepared in 5 minutes.

Ingredients:

A frozen banana that has been peeled and cut into chunks
1 cup of frozen strawberries
2 tbsp. flaxseed meal
1 cup low-fat vanilla almond milk.

Method:

1. Pour the banana, strawberry, flaxseed meal, and almond milk into a blender.
2. Blend until it forms a smooth puree.
3. Nutritional facts: The drink contains about 273 calories, 7.8 grams of protein, 47.1 grams of carbohydrates, 8.2 grams of fat, and 221.1 mg of sodium.

FLAX AND SUNFLOWER SEED BREAD

Children have always been lovers of bread and other products. This flax and sunflower seed bread is particularly good for seed lovers and tasty enough for children to enjoy. The process for the bread preparation is usually within 10 minutes while the bread itself is cooked for 30 minutes or more depending on the size of the bread in servings.

Ingredients:

1⅓ Bob's Red Mill 1 tol Gluten Free Baking Mix
One teaspoon of salt
1 tsp active dry yeast
¼ cup flaxseed½ cup of sunflower seeds

Method:

1. Put all the ingredients (except the sunflower seeds) in the pan in the bread machine. Add the sunflower seeds only after the kneading process had been completed.

Nutritional facts: 140 calories, 4.2 grams of protein, 22.7 grams of carbo-hydrate, 4.2 grams of fat, 4.1 mg of cholesterol, 168.6 mg of sodium.

PUMPKIN PROTEIN COOKIES

These pumpkin protein cookies are particularly excellent for breakfast and are like those in the store. The cookies contain a lot of protein which will help keep your child full. Furthermore, the snacks are sugar-free, thereby helping your child deal with Tourette's syndrome or Tics. For 14 servings of pumpkin protein cookies, you're likely to spend about an estimated 20 minutes.

Ingredients:

¾ cup of Allulose granular
1 cup rolled oats
1½ Bob's Red Mill 1 tol Gluten Free Baking Mix
1¾ teaspoons baking powder
½ teaspoon salt
2 teaspoons ground cinnamon
1 teaspoon ground nutmeg
½ cup pumpkin puree
1 tsp. avocado oil
2 teaspoons water
egg whites
1 teaspoon molasses1 teaspoon flaxseed

Method:

1. Heat the oven to about 175 °C.
2. Whisk the Allulose oats, gluten-free flour, baking soda, baking powder, cinnamon, salt, and nutmeg.
3. You should add in the pumpkin, avocado oil, water, molasses, and egg whites. After this is done, you could add the flaxseeds, roll the dough into 14 balls, and arrange it on a baking sheet.
4. After this is done, all you need to do is place it in the oven and bake for 5 minutes. It is important not to overbake those cookies; else, they will come out dried.

Nutritional facts: This serving contains 85 calories; 4.2 grams of protein; 13.1 grams of carbohydrate; 2.2 g of fat; 280 4.1 mg of sodium.

ALMOND FLOUR BREAD

Almond flour bread is a delicious bread made from almonds, high in protein and low in carbohydrates. The bread can be prepared in 55 minutes and would be in eight servings.

Ingredients:

1½ cups of almond flour
⅓ cup of flaxseed meal
4 eggs
2 tablespoons of olive oil
2 teaspoons baking powder
½ teaspoon salt
¼ cup unsweetened almond milk

Method:

1. Slightly grease the pan for the bread and preheat the oven to 175 °C.
2. Once this is done, mix the flaxseed meal, almond flour, almond milk, olive oil, eggs, salt, and baking powder in a bowl to get a smooth dough.
3. Put the mixed ingredients in the already greased loaf pan and place them in the preheated oven.
4. Although the entire process takes up to 55 minutes, the baking should only be for 40 minutes. Once the top of the bread turns golden brown, it means the bread is ready and should be transferred to a wire rack to cool for about 10 minutes.

HIGH-FIBRE, HIGH PROTEIN BREAKFAST BARS

This recipe can be prepared in 1 hour 45 minutes and can produce at least 12 bars.

Ingredients:

Cooking spray
1½ cups quick-cooking oats
¼ cup wheat germ
¼ cup ground flaxseed
2 tbsp. vanilla flavored hemp protein powder
1 tbsp. ground cinnamon
½ teaspoon salt
3 bananas
¼ cup peanut butter
2 tbsp. honey
1 teaspoon vanilla extract
¼ cup of natural peanut butter

Method:

1. The oven is first preheated to about 190 °C and line a 8* 8-inch baking dish with aluminum foil, hanging across the sides of the pan.
2. After this is done, the pan needs to be sprayed with cooking spray.
3. Then you stir the flax seed, protein powder, salt, cinnamon, wheat germ together in a container to make a dough.
4. You mash the bananas in another bowl and add peanuts, honey, and vanilla extract into the squashed banana.
5. Stir the ingredients well and allow them to settle to make a banana mixture.
6. Spread the mixture into the lined baking dish.
7. Bake the mixture in the preheated oven for at least 20 minutes and spread ¼ cup of peanut butter over the top of the dough while baking.
8. Continue to bake the dough until the edges of the dough become lightly brown at the edges and leave for 10 minutes to cool down.
9. Allow the bread to cool in the pan and lift it out with the bars of the aluminum foil as the handles.
10. Cut it into different sizes and wrap it in plastic wrap before storing it in the refrigerator.
11. You must use the hemp protein powder because it has the highest fiber present in it. This recipe contains 169 calories, 2 grams of protein, 21.3 grams of carbohydrates, 7.6 grams of fat, and 148 mg of sodium.

BRAN FLAX MUFFINS

These bran flax muffins are oatmeal muffins with carrots, raisins, nuts, and apples. The muffins are low in fat, rich in fiber, and extremely delicious, appealing to small children. These can be prepared within 35 minutes and make a serving of 15 muffins.

Ingredients:

1½ cups Bob's Red Mill 1 tol Gluten Free Baking Mix
¾ cup ground flaxseed
1 cup brown sugar
¾ cup oat bran
2 tsp baking soda
2 teaspoons baking soda
2 eggs
2 tablespoons of vegetable oil
1 teaspoon of vanilla extract
2 shredded and peeled apples
1 cup of chopped nuts
½ cup of raisins

Method:

1. Preheat the oven up to 175 ºC and grease a muffin pan with paper muffin liners.
2. Mix the flaxseed ingredients, baking soda, baking powder, cinnamon, salt, and brown sugar in a big bowl until it forms a dough.
3. Add the milk, vanilla, oil, and eggs together until they're properly blended.
4. Later introduce the carrots, apples, nuts, and raisins and stir them properly.
5. Fill up the prepared muffin cups with the blended fruit mixture.
6. Bake the filled muffins at a temperature of 175 ºC for at least 15 minutes and a maximum of 20 minutes.
7. Place a toothpick within the muffin at the center to see if it is done within the time.

Nutritional facts: Each muffin contains 272 calories, 6.7 grams of protein, 40.9 grams of carbohydrates, 11 grams of fat, 25 mg of cholesterol, and 448.8 mg of sodium.

FLAXSEED CRACKERS

If flaxseed is mixed with the same volume of water, soaked and spread thin, you will get a nice cracker as a snack. These flaxseed crackers provide a healthy, nutty, tasty, and earthy snack. The snack is light, sturdy, perfect for dips, and can be tried with various healthy syrups. This will make it exciting for children and healthy for them while providing them with the required energy. The snacks take a long period to prepare but cook for only three hours.

Ingredients:

¾tsp. of salt
¼ tsp. of onion powder
¼ tsp. of garlic powder
1 cup of raw flaxseeds
1 cup of cold water1 pinch cayenne powder

Method:

1. The flaxseeds are placed in a bowl and are mixed with onion powder, garlic powder, cayenne, and salt.
2. Add water to the mixture and stir while it is covered with plastic wrap.
3. The mixture is kept in a refrigerator throughout the night.
4. The oven is preheated to 200 degrees, lined with a rimmed baking sheet, and covered with silicon parchment.
5. Move the soaked flaxseeds onto the baking sheets.
6. Use a spatula to spread the flaxseed into a thin rectangle, about ⅛ inches thick.
7. Cut out the rectangles into 32 small rectangles for shape.
8. Bake the content in the preheated oven for about 3 hours till it is dark and contracted.
9. Let the baked dough cool by leaving the door of the oven open.
10. To get the best from the flaxseeds, they should be soaked to ensure that they are completely digestible, and you can access their immense nutrients. You could use a flaxseed meal if you are unable to use raw flaxseed.
11. The crackers tend to lose their crispness after a day or so. You can simply dry them again in the oven to crisp them back up.

Nutritional facts: This cracker contains 104 calories, 3.6 grams of protein, 5.7 grams of carbohydrates, 8.2 grams of fat, and 224.8 mg of sodium.

HOMEMADE FLAXSEED MILK

If you are a parent that wants your child to eat healthy without breaking the bank and avoid chemicals and additives, then homemade flaxseed milk is perfect for your child. By reducing the amount of water used, you can have a thicker paste instead of creams while making your drink. This milk drink can be made within 20 minutes and should make up at least four servings.

Ingredients:

½ cup of flaxseeds
4½ cups of water

Method:

1. Put flax seeds and water together in a blender and blend very fast for a minute; take a rest for about 2 minutes and blend again on a high for a minute; take a break for 5 minutes again and blend for 30 seconds.
2. Add milk through a nut bag or a filter lined with cheesecloth in a pitcher or glass container.
3. Press the flaxseed pulp to the back of the spoon to get the liquid out.
4. Get the cheesecloth around the solids to extract the liquid.

You must store the drink in a tight container and in the refrigerator for three days. You should also shake the container well before use because of the drink's gelling effect. The flaxseed pulp, the solid extract, can also be used in other gluten-free recipes.

Nutritional facts: The drink contains 3.5g of protein, 5.6g of calories, 13.8mg of sodium, 8.2g of fat, and 104 calories.

A note on energy foods

Legumes, peas, and cranberries are healthy, nutritious, and full of good carbohydrates, providing children with all the energy they need to remain active throughout the day. The importance of these recipes cannot be overemphasized and knowing how to prepare them for your child becomes imperative.

QUINOA SALAD WITH KALE, CRANBERRIES, AND MINT

It's easy to source mint in almost every garden in spring. If you love adding it to your salad, then this quinoa salad is a healthy and nutritious option.

Tips

Rinsing: Rinse the quinoa before cooking it to remove the coatings that make it bitter when cooked. You could use a mesh to sieve off the coatings after each use.

Know the appropriate water-to-quinoa ratio: Most people say that two cups of water for a cup of quinoa would suffice. However, quinoa tastes better with less water.

Make use of tricolor or red quinoa: The texture of the red quinoa is usually firmer and is better for salads.

Substitutes:

- If you can't get the tricolor or red color quinoa, you could always use the normal or brown quinoa.
- You can use avocado for more vegetables or spinach or arugula instead of kale.
- Spice it up by adding roasted pecans and walnuts or add some cheese such as goat's cheese or feta.

Ingredients:

1⅔ cups of water for a cup of red or tricolored quinoa
1 cup of chopped kale
2 tbsp. of extra olive oil
1 large lemon
1 medium scallion
½ tsp lemon zest
⅓ cup chopped fresh spearmint leaves
¾ tsp. of kosher salt
⅓ cup of dried cranberries

Method:

1. Mix the water and the salt together in a saucepan and boil over high heat.
2. Reduce the heat, add quinoa, cover the mixture and allow to simmer for about 18 to 20 minutes till the liquid has been absorbed.
3. Check the quinoa with a fork and put it aside for it to cool.

4. Immediately after the quinoa has cooled, add kale, dried cranberries, lemon zest, scallions, olive oil, and lemon juice.
5. Keep the food in the refrigerator till you are ready to eat and serve.

INSTANT POT REFRIED BEANS

These instant pot refried beans are an easy fat-free food that can be cooked in a single pot and are a healthy Mexican meal for the whole family. Most refried beans are cooked twice to get the desired effect; however, instant pot refried beans can be easily made by cooking pinto beans until they are tender and mashing them until they are creamy. The beans can be refrigerated and eaten as leftovers with tacos and burritos.

I use pinto beans when making this recipe because they are sweeter, earthy in flavor, and tender. If you can't find the pinto beans, you could easily use black beans instead.

Ingredients:

2 cups pinto beans
3 cups of water
½ yellow onions
1tsp of ground cumin
2 cloves of garlic
1tsp of chili powder
¼ tsp of ground black pepper
½ or ¾ tsp of fine sea salt
A pinch of cayenne pepperFresh cilantro and lime wedges (optional)

Method:

1. Add the drained beans, water, garlic, and onions together in an instant pot.
2. Stir the beans well until submerged in the liquid and cover the lid to make it airtight.
3. Cook in the pressure pot for 20 minutes.
4. Once the cooking is complete, let the pressure out naturally for 10 minutes and move the valve to 'vent' to release the pressure. When the valve drops, take away the lid and drain the beans while you keep the liquid.
5. Transfer the cooked beans back into the pot and add cumin, black pepper and chilli peppers, salt, and cayenne pepper.
6. Mash the beans with the potato masher to make them smooth or blend them to achieve a puree.
7. Add more salt and seasoning to the beans and serve warm with cilantro and lime juice added to taste.
8. You could store the leftovers for a week in the fridge in an airtight container.

Chapter 17

Personalized Tracker

Throughout this book, tons of information has been thrown at you and you may be finding it difficult to know where to start. Trust me, I have been in this position, and I understand. The information received is so enormous that it becomes cumbersome for you to even begin. I wanted to make it as easy as possible for you, so I wrote down how I started. I hope that this personalized plan will help guide you on your journey and support you and your child to reduce Tics or Tourette's symptoms.

Tic symptoms can be reduced and managed through developing a healthy lifestyle focusing on areas such as rest, stress management, exercise, and diet. These steps must be taken every day and adjusted to fit into your schedule and lifestyle.

I have included my trigger tracker for you so that you can start tracking your child's day right away.

You can use the version at the end of this chapter or, if you have the eBook version of this book, *download your own printable **HERE**.: https://www.dropbox.com/s/kho2d8rt7mjviea/Trigger%20Tracker%20Journal.pdf?dl=0*

Here is a little guidance on the best way to fill this out. Please be as detailed as possible as this is going to be our investigative journal. Keeping a tracking journal will create an enjoyable positive habit and give us clues into what might be going on.

1. Enter your meals every day and be detailed about what you eat. If it goes in your mouth or your child's mouth, it goes on this sheet.
2. Track all your supplements daily, make sure to include names and dosages.
3. Poop? This is not a yes or no question. Write down the details (constipation, diarrhea, color, texture). Gross? Yes! There are clues in the poo.
4. Mood - details, details, details! How were you feeling? Did your mood fluctuate, were you tired, wired, etc...

5. Did you move today? Tell me what you did for exercise today.
6. How was your sleep? Like a rock, tossed and turned, got up to pee 50 times, woke up at 2 am and couldn't go back to sleep. You get the idea!
7. List any other symptoms, toxin exposure, or other details.
8. Finally, you can tell me about your day overall.

Feel free to print as many of the journal pages as you like. You may also edit this journal daily in Adobe Acrobat if it is available to you and you have the eBook version of this book.

Remember that this is a marathon and not a sprint. It is going to take time to heal the body and get back on the healthy path.

MEALS:

1.

2.

3.

Snacks:

SUPPLEMENTS:

a.m.

p.m.

POOP:

MOOD:

ACTIVITY:

SLEEP:

ADDITIONAL SYMPTOMS/TOXINS:

WAS IT A GOOD DAY?

WWW.REGENERATING.HEALTH

References

www.mofga.org/resources/health/neurological-disorders

www.healthline.com/health/gut-health#the-takeaway

www.brainharmony.com/blog/2020/12/5/why-tics-happen-and-how-to-fix-them

www.medicalnewstoday.com/articles/326575

www.pubmed.ncbi.nlm.nih.gov/29268618

www.livestrong.com/article/486014-supplements-for-tics-tourettes/kidshealth.org/en/parents/medical

www.additudemag.com/screener-tic-disorder-symptoms-test-children

www.theatlantic.com/health/archive/2014/03/the-toxins-that-threaten-our-brains/284466

www.nhs.uk/mental-health/feelings-symptoms-behaviours/feelings-and-symptoms/anxiety-fear-panic

www.nhs.uk/live-well/sleep-and-tiredness/healthy-sleep-tips-for-children

www.nhs.uk/live-well/sleep-and-tiredness/how-much-sleep-do-kids-need

www.webmd.com/balance/stress-management/stress-management

www.cincinnatichildrens.org/health/t/tics-ts-meds

www.allrecipes.com/recipe/18010/flax-and-sunflower-seed-bread

www.allrecipes.com/recipe/50441/pumpkin-protein-cookies

www.allrecipes.com/recipe/246002/almond-flour-bread

www.allrecipes.com/recipe/231925/high-fiber-high-protein-breakfast-bars

www.webmd.com/balance/stress-management/stress-management

www.allrecipes.com/recipes/17642/ingredients/nuts-and-seeds/flax-seeds

www.allrecipes.com/recipe/16877/bran-flax-muffins

www.allrecipes.com/recipe/261801/flax-seed-crackers

www.allrecipes.com/recipe/161325/flax-seed-smoothie

www.allrecipes.com/recipe/245438/homemade-flax-seed-milk

www.skinnytaste.com/quinoa-salad-with-kale-cranberries-and-mint

www.skinnytaste.com/refried-beans

www.skinnytaste.com/black-bean-tacos

About the Author

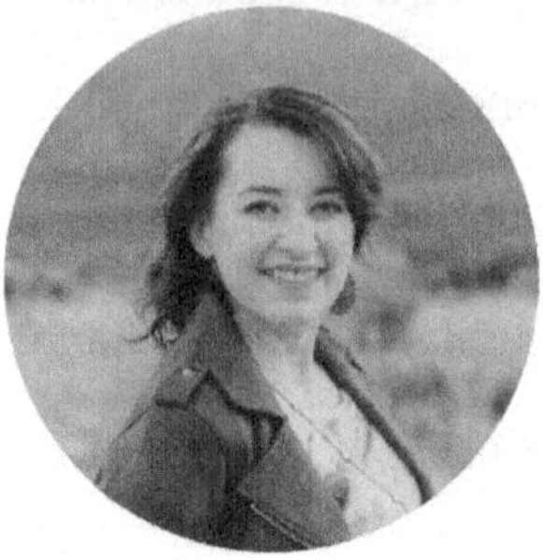

Dr. Piper Gibson, DFM, AHND, TND, BCDNM is a Doctor of Functional Medicine, Doctor of Advanced Holistic Nutrition, a Traditional Naturopathic Doctor, and is a Board-Certified Doctor of Natural Medicine. Piper helps scared, frustrated, and overwhelmed parents get access to the tools and resources they need so they can start to reduce their child's Tic disorder symptoms naturally.

She is the founder of Regenerating Health and has been able to help many families all over the world to gain control of their child's neurodevelopmental issues using food, functional lab testing, and natural approaches.

She resides in New Mexico with her husband and two sons. When she isn't working in the health space you can find her relaxing at the lake with her family.

If you are interested in working with Piper and her team you can connect at *www.regenerating.health*

Social Media:

Facebook: *http://www.facebook.com/RegeneratingHealth*
Instagram: *http://www.instagram.com/regeneratinghealth*

GAD 1 SNP Glutamate Guide

Ingredients that always contain processed free glutamic acid:

Glutamic Acid (E 620), Glutamate (E 620) Monosodium Glutamate (E 621), Monopotassium Glutamate (E 622), Calcium Glutamate (E 623), Monoammonium Glutamate (E 624), Magnesium Glutamate (E 625), Natrium Glutamate, Yeast Extract, Anything "hydrolyzed", Any "hydrolyzed protein", Calcium Caseinate, Sodium Caseinate, Yeast Food, Yeast Nutrient, Autolyzed Yeast, Gelatin, Textured Protein, Soy Protein, Soy Protein Concentrate, Soy Protein Isolate, Whey Protein, Whey Protein Concentrate, Whey Protein Isolate, Anything "...protein", Vetsin, Ajinomoto

Ingredients that often contain or produce processed free glutamic acid:

Carrageenan (E 407), Bouillon, and broth stock. Any "flavors" or "flavoring, Maltodextrin, Citric acid, Citrate (E 330), anything "ultra-pasteurized", Barley malt, Pectin (E 440), Protease, anything "enzyme modified", anything containing "enzymes", Malt Extract, Soy sauce, Soy sauce extract, anything "protein-fortified", anything "fermented", Seasonings

The following are ingredients suspected of containing or creating processed free glutamic acid and may be an MSG-reaction trigger in HIGHLY SENSITIVE people:

Corn starch, Corn syrup, Modified food starch, Lipolyzed butterfat, Dextrose, Rice syrup, Brown rice syrup, Milk powder, Reduced fat milk (skim; 1%; 2%), Most things labeled "Low Fat" or "No Fat", Anything labeled "Enriched" Anything labeled "Vitamin Enriched".

Made in the USA
Monee, IL
04 November 2026

67385552R10075